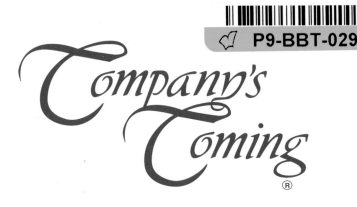

# Healthy In A Hurry

*Jean Paré*

**www.companyscoming.com**
visit our website

## Front Cover

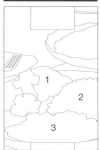

1. Honey Ginger
   Salmon, page 93
2. Fragrant Rice,
   page 134
3. Tropical Peppers,
   page 124

Props courtesy of:
   Casa Bugatti
   The Bay

## Back Cover

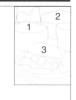

1. Apple Carrot Slaw,
   page 37
2. Creamy Pasta Salad,
   page 44
3. Mushroom Steak
   Sandwiches, page 69

Props courtesy of: Danesco Inc.
Anchor Hocking
Canada.

**Healthy In A Hurry**

Copyright © Company's Coming Publishing Limited

Third Printing April 2010

**Library and Archives Canada Cataloguing in Publication**
Paré, Jean, date
Healthy in a hurry / Jean Paré.
(Original series)
Includes index.
At head of title: Company's Coming.
ISBN 978-1-897069-96-7
1. Quick and easy cookery. I. Title. II. Series: Paré, Jean, date-
Original series.
TX833.5.P349 2009    641.5'55    C2008-903775-8

Published by
**Company's Coming Publishing Limited**
2311 – 96 Street
Edmonton, Alberta, Canada T6N 1G3
Tel: 780-450-6223   Fax: 780-450-1857
www.companyscoming.com

Company's Coming is a registered trademark owned by Company's Coming Publishing Limited

We acknowledge the financial support of the Government of Canada through the Book Publishing Industry Development Program (BPIDP) for our publishing activities.

Printed in China

We gratefully acknowledge the following suppliers for their generous support of our Test and Photography Kitchens:

*Broil King Barbecues*
*Corelle®*
*Hamilton Beach® Canada*
*Lagostina®*
*Proctor Silex® Canada*
*Tupperware®*

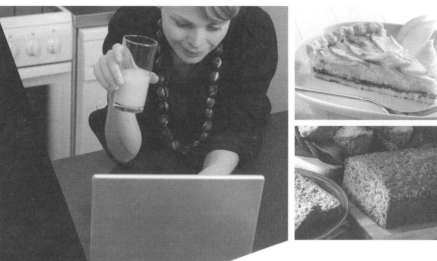

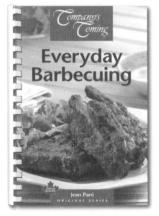
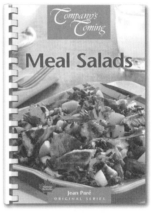
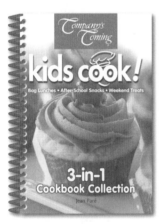
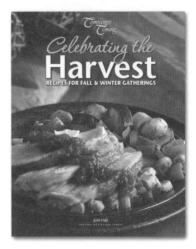

# Table of Contents

# The Company's Coming Story

Jean Paré (pronounced "jeen PAIR-ee") grew up understanding that the combination of family, friends and home cooking is the best recipe for a good life. From her mother, she learned to appreciate good cooking, while her father praised even her earliest attempts in the kitchen. When Jean left home, she took with her a love of cooking, many family recipes and an intriguing desire to read cookbooks as if they were novels!

*"Never share a recipe you wouldn't use yourself."*

When her four children had all reached school age, Jean volunteered to cater the 50th anniversary celebration of the Vermilion School of Agriculture, now Lakeland College, in Alberta, Canada. Working out of her home, Jean prepared a dinner for more than 1,000 people, launching a flourishing catering operation that continued for over 18 years. During that time, she had countless opportunities to test new ideas with immediate feedback—resulting in empty plates and contented customers! Whether preparing cocktail sandwiches for a house party or serving a hot meal for 1,500 people, Jean Paré earned a reputation for great food, courteous service and reasonable prices.

As requests for her recipes increased, Jean was often asked the question, "Why don't you write a cookbook?" Jean responded by teaming up with her son, Grant Lovig, in the fall of 1980 to form Company's Coming Publishing Limited. The publication of *150 Delicious Squares* on April 14, 1981 marked the debut of what would soon become one of the world's most popular cookbook series.

The company has grown since those early days when Jean worked from a spare bedroom in her home. Today, she continues to write recipes while working closely with the staff of the Recipe Factory, as the Company's Coming test kitchen is affectionately known.

There she fills the role of mentor, assisting with the development of recipes people most want to use for everyday cooking and easy entertaining. Every Company's Coming recipe is *kitchen-tested* before it is approved for publication.

Jean's daughter, Gail Lovig, is responsible for marketing and distribution, leading a team that includes sales personnel located in major cities across Canada. Company's Coming cookbooks are distributed in Canada, the United States, Australia and other world markets. Bestsellers many times over in English, Company's Coming cookbooks have also been published in French and Spanish.

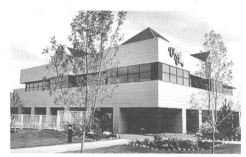

Familiar and trusted in home kitchens around the world, Company's Coming cookbooks are offered in a variety of formats. Highly regarded as kitchen workbooks, the softcover Original Series, with its lay-flat plastic comb binding, is still a favourite among readers.

Jean Paré's approach to cooking has always called for *quick and easy recipes* using *everyday ingredients*. That view has served her well. The recipient of many awards, including the Queen Elizabeth Golden Jubilee Medal, Jean was appointed Member of the Order of Canada, her country's highest lifetime achievement honour.

Jean continues to gain new supporters by adhering to what she calls The Golden Rule of Cooking: *Never share a recipe you wouldn't use yourself.* It's an approach that has worked—*millions of times over!*

# Foreword

For many of us, the thought of preparing a meal that's healthy and quick is a contradiction in terms. We think wholesome eating means lots of scrubbing, peeling and slow cooking, while fast food can only equal high levels of fat, salt and sugar. How is it possible to put speed and nutrition on one plate?

Easy, with *Healthy in a Hurry*. Every one of our nourishing recipes can be on the table in 30 minutes or less—and that includes the preparation and cooking times!

Our secret? We've used many commercially prepped ingredients, such as frozen veggies, fresh stir-fry vegetable mixes and ready-sliced beef strips, to help get you in and out of the kitchen fast. And while we've pared down ingredients for each recipe, we've carefully selected high-impact flavour boosters—balsamic vinegar, citrus juices, zests, low-sodium broth, no-salt seasoning and sesame oil, for example—to make each dish a success.

To help you use your time effectively, we'll occasionally nudge you along to the next step of a recipe even as it's simmering on the stove or baking in the oven. We'll also share our time-saving tips on everything from shopping to freezing, so meal-planning can become an effortless part of your life.

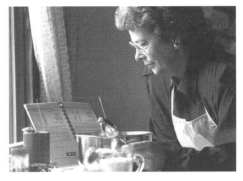

We've worked hard to cut down the sodium and fat in these dishes, while pumping up the flavour. And we've scattered extra health-related tips and facts through the book as FYIs.

*Healthy in a Hurry* has nutritious suggestions from breakfast and brunch to dinner and desserts. Surprising but delicious ingredient combinations will please family and friends.

Once you've tried a few of our recipes, you'll see that fast, nutritious food doesn't have to be an impossible contradiction. It's easy to get *Healthy in a Hurry!*

*Jean Paré*

## Nutrition Information Guidelines

Each recipe is analyzed using the most current version of the Canadian Nutrient File from Health Canada, which is based on the United States Department of Agriculture (USDA) Nutrient Database.

- If more than one ingredient is listed (such as "butter or hard margarine"), or if a range is given (1 – 2 tsp., 5 – 10 mL), only the first ingredient or first amount is analyzed.

- For meat, poultry and fish, the serving size per person is based on the recommended 4 oz. (113 g) uncooked weight (without bone), which is 2 – 3 oz. (57 – 85 g) cooked weight (without bone)—approximately the size of a deck of playing cards.

- Milk used is 1% M.F. (milk fat), unless otherwise stated.

- Cooking oil used is canola oil, unless otherwise stated.

- Ingredients indicating "sprinkle," "optional," or "for garnish" are not included in the nutrition information.

- The fat in recipes and combination foods can vary greatly depending on the sources and types of fats used in each specific ingredient. For these reasons, the amount of saturated, monounsaturated and polyunsaturated fats may not add up to the total fat content.

Vera C. Mazurak, Ph.D.
Nutritionist

# Keeping it Healthy
# When You're in a Hurry

## Perfect your planning

Sorry to say, but the biggest time-saver is the one people have the hardest time with—planning. Avoid the daily routine of staring into your refrigerator, hoping for inspiration, and take the few extra minutes a week needed to make mealtime a breeze.

- **Have a running grocery list.** Get a magnetic shopping list and place it on your fridge. When you run low on something, or feel a little bit inspired, add the necessary ingredients to the list.

- **Plan your meals a week in advance.** This will make grocery shopping a snap. Just check the recipes to make sure you have everything you need. After all, there's nothing worse than getting halfway through a recipe and realizing you're missing an essential ingredient!

- **Take meat out the night before to thaw in the fridge.** The benefits of this are twofold: you won't be tempted to opt for takeout when you know you have something waiting to be cooked up; and you won't have to deal with those rubbery edges that mysteriously appear when you defrost meat in the microwave.

- **Double recipes and freeze extras.** Make a big dish and then freeze the leftovers in meal-sized portions that you can quickly heat up when you're extra low on time.

- **Double staple ingredients and freeze extras.** Consider cooking up extra ground beef, ground chicken, beans, rice and whole grains. They freeze well and, because they are already cooked, will help to reduce the cooking times of any future recipes.

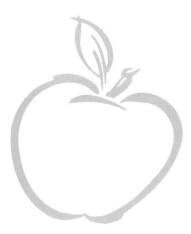

- **Stock up on often-used ingredients.** Whole wheat pasta, prepackaged low-sodium stock, rice and your favourite spices should all be at the ready when you're ready to cook.

## Fighting the snack attack

When you're on the go and hunger hits, it's easy to surrender and give in to the allure of the junk food counter of your nearest convenience store. But fear not, it's unlikely you'll have to raise a white flag if you have prepared, healthy snacks on hand.

Prepare your snacks at home, put them in individual baggies and have them waiting in your fridge when you need to grab-and-go. Or you can buy healthy prepackaged snacks in the produce or dairy section of your local grocer's. And don't underestimate the convenience of buying prewashed baby carrots and sugar snap peas—no fuss, no muss, just pop them in a baggie and your snack is ready. Consider the following foods as potential snack items in your battle against processed, fatty junk food.

- 100% fruit leather
- 100% juice boxes
- Applesauce
- Bottled water
- Dried fruit (raisins, apricots, apples, prunes)
- Individual portions of low-fat cheese
- Low-fat yogurt & cottage cheese
- Pre-cut fruit
- Pre-cut veggies
- Raw nuts & seeds (almonds, sunflower seeds, peanuts)
- Rice cakes & baked rice crackers
- Soy nuts (in smaller amounts)
- Whole-grain crackers

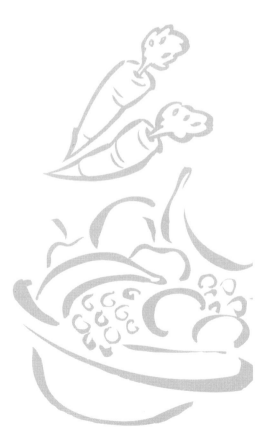

## Making it faster with freezer fare

Your freezer can be your best friend when trying to plan and serve healthy meals—because, really, all you have to do is reheat. Stackable plastic containers and sealable freezer bags are your best options when freezing food. Remove as much air as possible from freezer bags to keep your food at its optimum freshness, but leave some space in rigid plastic containers to allow for expansion. Be sure to label each container with the contents and the date you froze it. No one wants to eat the "mystery meat" or the "dinner surprise!"

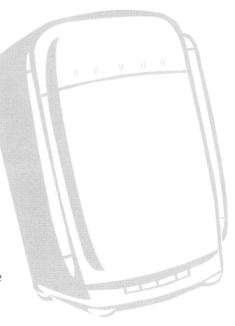

When adding food to your freezer, be sure to rotate so the oldest food is on the top—this way you won't be able to forget about it if it's in plain view. Freezing does keep food safe for quite awhile, but the quality of the taste will decrease over time.

## Learning to love the light

Shaving off a little bit of fat here and a few calories there will add up to big health benefits over time. Consider this: if you use reduced-fat ranch dressing, you'll save 40 calories and 5 grams of total fat per tablespoon;

and if you use fat-free ranch dressing, you'll save 56 calories and 7 grams of total fat per tablespoon! By the end of the year you'll have cut out literally thousands of calories in salad dressing alone!

Healthy eating does not have to take longer. It can be done simply by shopping smarter. Easily cut down on fat and calories by trying the reduced-fat or lighter versions of favourite foods—sometimes you can't even taste the difference!

Embrace this philosophy when buying meats as well. Trim the fat off your meat before cooking. Use leaner cuts, poultry without skin and white meat instead of dark. Choose deli meats less often—but when you do, choose leaner meats with less sodium.

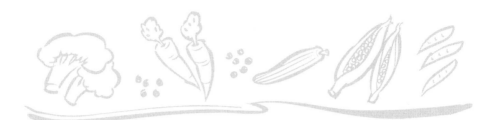

## Taking it a step further

So, now that you've got the right ingredients and the right recipes, are there any other ways you can make your cooking healthier? You bet! Just follow some of the tips below and apply them in your cooking whenever possible.

- To retain more nutrients, steam or microwave vegetables instead of boiling them.

- Use non-stick cookware to minimize your use of oil or margarine.

- Use whole-wheat pasta, bread and tortillas and brown or wild rice in your meals.

- If you're concerned about sodium, don't add salt in the preparation stages of cooking. Many ingredients already have salt added to them including condiments, canned and dried soups and seasonings. Make healthier meals by using reduced-sodium products or substitutes.

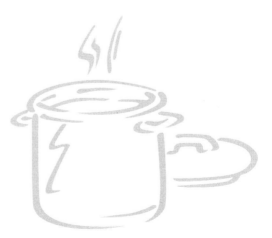

# Blast O' Berry Smoothie

*Get your morning blast o' energy from this creamy, purple smoothie full of refreshing tropical flavours.*

| | | |
|---|---|---|
| Chopped papaya | 2 cups | 500 mL |
| Frozen (or fresh) blueberries | 2 cups | 500 mL |
| Peach mango dessert tofu | 10 2/3 oz. | 300 g |
| Pineapple juice | 1 cup | 250 mL |
| Low-fat plain yogurt | 1/2 cup | 125 mL |

Process all 5 ingredients in blender or food processor until smooth. Makes about 6 cups (1.5 L). Serves 4.

*1 serving:* 164 Calories; 2.3 g Total Fat (0.2 g Mono, trace Poly, 0.5 g Sat); 2 mg Cholesterol; 35 g Carbohydrate; 4 g Fibre; 5 g Protein; 30 mg Sodium

# Mango Tango

*Get your morning energy boost in a convenient beverage! Using frozen fruit helps to thicken and chill smoothies. For a more intense mango flavour, use mango nectar or mango-peach fruit cocktail instead of orange juice.*

| | | |
|---|---|---|
| Frozen mango pieces | 2 cups | 500 mL |
| Milk (or soy milk) | 1 cup | 250 mL |
| Peach (or peach-mango) dessert tofu | 5 1/3 oz. | 150 g |
| Orange juice | 1/2 cup | 125 mL |
| Wheat germ, toasted (see Tip, page 13) | 1 tbsp. | 15 mL |

Process all 5 ingredients in blender until smooth. Makes 3 1/2 cups (875 mL). Serves 2.

*1 serving:* 254 Calories; 3.5 g Total Fat (0.7 g Mono, 0.3 g Poly, 1.1 g Sat); 8 mg Cholesterol; 52 g Carbohydrate; 4 g Fibre; 9 g Protein; 74 mg Sodium

# Cranberry Oatmeal

*Oatmeal doesn't have to be boring! We've jazzed up this version with the tangy taste of cranberry. Just add milk or sprinkle a few toasted almonds over the top for a delicious breakfast that's also a good source of fibre.*

| | | |
|---|---|---|
| Cranberry cocktail | 2 cups | 500 mL |
| Water | 1 cup | 250 mL |
| Salt | 1/4 tsp. | 1 mL |
| Quick-cooking rolled oats | 1 1/3 cups | 325 mL |
| Dried cranberries | 1/2 cup | 125 mL |

Combine first 3 ingredients in medium saucepan. Bring to a boil.

Add oats and cranberries. Stir. Cook on medium for 3 to 5 minutes, stirring occasionally, until thickened. Remove from heat. Cover. Let stand for 5 minutes. Makes about 3 cups (750 mL).

*1 cup (250 mL): 306 Calories; 3.2 g Total Fat (0.1 g Mono, 0.2 g Poly, trace Sat); 0 mg Cholesterol; 66 g Carbohydrate; 5 g Fibre; 6 g Protein; 199 mg Sodium*

**Variation:** Instead of cranberry cocktail and dried cranberries, use the same amounts of your favourite fruit juice blend and a dried fruit to complement. Peach-mango cocktail with chopped dried apricot makes a great combination.

 To toast wheat germ, spread evenly in an ungreased frying pan. Heat and stir on medium until golden. To bake, spread evenly in an ungreased shallow pan. Bake in a 350°F (175°C) oven for 3 minutes, stirring or shaking often, until golden. Cool before adding to recipe.

# Breakfast Bites

*Cookies for breakfast? Not quite, but these bites are quick and easy to make. Healthy whether eaten as a breakfast, a dessert or a snack.*

| | | |
|---|---|---|
| Large egg, fork-beaten | 1 | 1 |
| Overripe medium banana, mashed | 1 | 1 |
| Grated carrot | 1 cup | 250 mL |
| Sliced natural almonds, toasted (see Tip, below) | 1/2 cup | 125 mL |
| Brown sugar, packed | 1/2 cup | 125 mL |
| Unsweetened applesauce | 1/4 cup | 60 mL |
| Vanilla extract | 1/4 tsp. | 1 mL |
| Whole-wheat flour | 1 cup | 250 mL |
| Quick-cooking rolled oats | 1/2 cup | 125 mL |
| Flaxseed | 1/4 cup | 60 mL |
| Baking soda | 1/2 tsp. | 2 mL |
| Salt | 1/2 tsp. | 2 mL |
| Ground cinnamon | 1/4 tsp. | 1 mL |

Combine first 7 ingredients in large bowl.

Add remaining 6 ingredients. Stir until no dry flour remains. Drop by rounded tablespoonfuls about 1 inch (2.5 cm) apart onto greased cookie sheet. Bake in 350°F (175°C) oven for about 12 minutes until set and bottoms are browned. Remove bites from cookie sheet and place on wire rack to cool. Makes 24 bites.

*1 bite: 74 Calories; 2.2 g Total Fat (0.9 g Mono, 0.9 g Poly, 0.2 g Sat); 8 mg Cholesterol; 12 g Carbohydrate; 2 g Fibre; 2 g Protein; 84 mg Sodium*

*tip* To toast nuts, seeds or coconut, place them in an ungreased shallow frying pan. Heat on medium for 3 to 5 minutes, stirring often, until golden. To bake, spread them evenly in an ungreased shallow pan. Bake in a 350°F (175°C) oven for 5 to 10 minutes, stirring or shaking often, until golden.

# Potato Kale Frittata

*Who doesn't love a one-dish meal? This hearty frittata has just enough spicy heat to put some pep in your early-morning step. This recipe can be easily halved and prepared in a medium-sized frying pan.*

| | | |
|---|---|---|
| Canola oil | 1 tbsp. | 15 mL |
| Diced peeled potato | 1 1/2 cups | 375 mL |
| Finely chopped onion | 2/3 cup | 150 mL |
| Garlic cloves, minced | 2 | 2 |
| (or 1/2 tsp., 2 mL, powder) | | |
| Dried crushed chilies | 1/2 tsp. | 2 mL |
| Finely chopped kale leaves, lightly packed | 3 cups | 750 mL |
| (see Tip, page 110) | | |
| Sun-dried tomato pesto | 1 tbsp. | 15 mL |
| Packages of low-cholesterol egg product | 2 | 2 |
| (8 oz., 227 mL, each), see Note | | |
| Grated Parmesan cheese | 1/4 cup | 60 mL |

Preheat broiler. Heat canola oil in large frying pan on medium. Add next 4 ingredients. Cook, covered, for about 8 minutes, stirring occasionally, until potato is browned and tender-crisp.

Add kale and pesto. Stir well. Cook, covered, for about 5 minutes, stirring occasionally, until kale is softened.

Pour egg product over kale mixture. Reduce heat to medium-low. Cook, covered, for 3 to 5 minutes until bottom is golden and top is almost set. Remove from heat. Sprinkle with Parmesan cheese. Broil on centre rack in oven for 3 to 5 minutes until golden and set (See Tip, page 22). Serves 4.

*1 serving: 224 Calories; 8.7 g Total Fat (4.0 g Mono, 1.5 g Poly, 2.3 g Sat); 100 mg Cholesterol; 18 g Carbohydrate; 2 g Fibre; 16 g Protein; 147 mg Sodium*

**Note:** Instead of using low-cholesterol egg product, use 8 large eggs, fork-beaten.

# Cinnamon Apple Grits

*You may not want to kiss these grits, but you'll probably want to kiss the cook who made them! This sunny yellow cornmeal mixture with an apple, raisin and walnut topping provides sweet relief from everyday oatmeal.*

| | | |
|---|---|---|
| Chopped, peeled cooking apple (such as McIntosh) | 1 1/2 cups | 375 mL |
| Frozen concentrated apple juice, thawed | 1 cup | 250 mL |
| Water | 1/2 cup | 125 mL |
| Golden raisins | 1/2 cup | 125 mL |
| Liquid honey | 2 tbsp. | 30 mL |
| Ground cinnamon | 1 tsp. | 5 mL |
| Water | 3 1/2 cups | 875 mL |
| Frozen concentrated apple juice, thawed | 1/2 cup | 125 mL |
| Salt | 1/2 tsp. | 2 mL |
| Yellow cornmeal | 1 cup | 250 mL |
| Coarsely chopped walnuts | 1/2 cup | 125 mL |

Combine first 6 ingredients in medium saucepan. Bring to a boil. Reduce heat to medium. Boil gently, uncovered, for 10 minutes.

Meanwhile, combine next 3 ingredients in large saucepan. Bring to a boil. Slowly add cornmeal, stirring constantly. Reduce heat to low. Cook for 3 to 5 minutes, stirring often, until thickened to consistency of soft porridge.

Add walnuts to apple mixture. Stir. Spoon cornmeal mixture into 4 individual serving bowls. Spoon apple mixture over top. Serves 4.

*1 serving: 517 Calories; 10.9 g Total Fat (1.5 g Mono, 7.5 g Poly, 1.1 g Sat); 0 mg Cholesterol; 103 g Carbohydrate; 5 g Fibre; 7 g Protein; 323 mg Sodium*

Pictured at right.

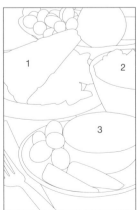

1. Double Strawberry Toast, page 20
2. Cinnamon Apple Grits, above
3. Sunny Tuscan Eggwiches, page 21

Props courtesy of: Pfaltzgraff Canada
                Anchor Hocking Canada
                Danesco Inc.

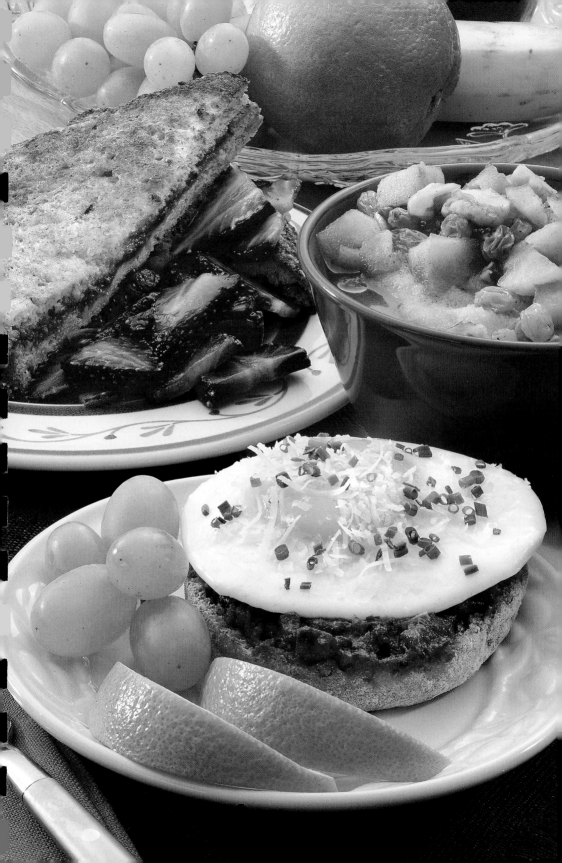

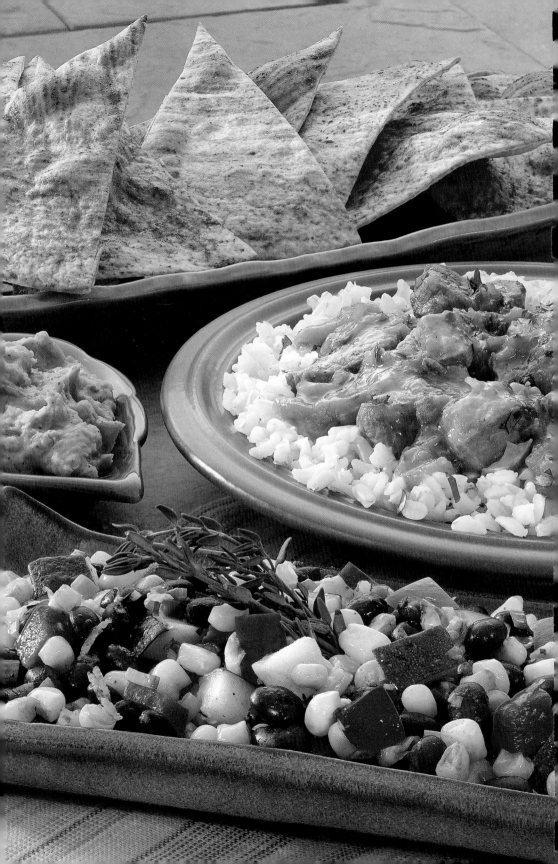

# Salmon Feta Frittata

*Easier than omelettes! Wow your nearest and dearest at your next brunch with this delicious salmon, onion and egg dish—complemented with Dijon mustard and feta cheese.*

| | | |
|---|---|---|
| Canola oil | 1 tbsp. | 15 mL |
| Large eggs | 6 | 6 |
| Milk | 1 1/3 cups | 325 mL |
| Dijon mustard | 1 tbsp. | 15 mL |
| Lemon pepper | 1/4 tsp. | 1 mL |
| Can of pink salmon, drained, skin and round bones removed | 6 1/2 oz. | 184 g |
| Crumbled light feta cheese | 1/4 cup | 60 mL |
| Chopped green onion | 2 tbsp. | 30 mL |

Preheat broiler. Heat canola oil in large frying pan on medium.

Meanwhile, whisk next 4 ingredients in medium bowl until combined. Pour into frying pan. Cook, uncovered, without stirring, for 5 minutes.

Sprinkle with remaining 3 ingredients. Cook, covered, for about 5 minutes until bottom is golden and top is almost set. Remove from heat. Broil on centre rack in oven for about 2 minutes until golden and set (see Tip, page 22). Serves 4.

*1 serving: 244 Calories; 14.2 g Total Fat (5.4 g Mono, 2.2 g Poly, 3.7 g Sat); 316 mg Cholesterol; 5 g Carbohydrate; trace Fibre; 24 g Protein; 471 mg Sodium*

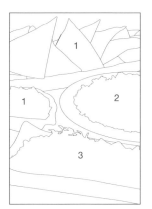

1. Tofu Bean Dip And Crisps, page 24
2. Apricot Jalapeño Pork, page 114
3. Black Bean And Corn Skillet, page 137

Props courtesy of: Out of the Fire Studio
The Bay

# Double Strawberry Toast

*Strawberries as far as the eye can see! These French toast sandwiches have strawberries inside and out. The honey, strawberry and lime topping adds that extra bit of delightful decadence.*

| | | |
|---|---|---|
| Liquid honey | 1/4 cup | 60 mL |
| Lime juice | 2 tbsp. | 30 mL |
| Grated lime zest | 1 tsp. | 5 mL |
| Sliced fresh strawberries | 3 cups | 750 mL |
| Package of low-cholesterol egg product (see Note) | 8 oz. | 227 mL |
| Vanilla soy milk | 1 cup | 250 mL |
| Coconut (or vanilla) extract | 1/2 tsp. | 2 mL |
| Strawberry jam | 2/3 cup | 150 mL |
| Whole-grain bread slices | 12 | 12 |
| Canola oil | 2 tbsp. | 30 mL |

Combine first 3 ingredients in medium bowl. Add strawberries. Stir well. Set aside.

Beat next 3 ingredients in large shallow bowl with a whisk until frothy. Set aside.

Spread about 1 1/2 tbsp. (25 mL) jam on 1 bread slice. Cover with second bread slice. Repeat with remaining jam and bread slices, making 6 sandwiches.

Heat 1 tbsp. (15 mL) canola oil in large frying pan on medium-low. Press one sandwich into egg mixture. Turn over to coat both sides. Transfer to frying pan. Repeat with 2 more sandwiches. Cook for about 4 minutes per side until golden. Transfer to serving platter. Keep warm in 200°F (95°C) oven. Repeat with remaining oil, sandwiches and egg mixture. Spoon 1/2 cup (125 mL) strawberry mixture over each sandwich. Serves 6.

*1 serving: 399 Calories; 8.6 g Total Fat (4.0 g Mono, 2.1 g Poly, 1.2 g Sat); 32 mg Cholesterol; 71 g Carbohydrate; 6 g Fibre; 12 g Protein; 336 mg Sodium*

Pictured on page 17.

**Note:** Instead of using low-cholesterol egg product, use 4 large eggs, fork-beaten.

# Sunny Tuscan Eggwiches

*Try the sunny side of Italy! Sun-dried tomato and balsamic flavours are a unique addition to a breakfast classic. The hand-held sandwich variation is easy to eat on the go. Excellent with a serving of fresh fruit.*

| | | |
|---|---|---|
| Whole-wheat English muffins, split | 2 | 2 |
| Sun-dried tomato pesto | 1/4 cup | 60 mL |
| Balsamic vinegar | 1 tbsp. | 15 mL |
| Dried crushed chilies | 1/4 tsp. | 1 mL |
| Olive (or canola) oil | 1 tsp. | 5 mL |
| Large eggs | 4 | 4 |
| Chopped fresh chives | 2 tbsp. | 30 mL |
| Grated Parmesan cheese | 1 tbsp. | 15 mL |

Toast English muffin halves in toaster until golden. Transfer to plate.

Meanwhile, combine next 3 ingredients in small bowl. Spoon mixture onto muffin halves. Set aside.

Heat olive oil in small frying pan on medium. Break eggs into pan. Cook, covered, for about 2 minutes until egg whites are just set and form a light film over yolk. Carefully place 1 egg over pesto mixture on each muffin half.

Sprinkle chives and Parmesan cheese over eggs. Makes 4 eggwiches.

*1 eggwich: 209 Calories; 10.5 g Total Fat (5.3 g Mono, 1.6 g Poly, 2.5 g Sat); 187 mg Cholesterol; 20 g Carbohydrate; 4 g Fibre; 11 g Protein; 363 mg Sodium*

Pictured on page 17.

**Variation:** To make these into hand-held sandwiches, cook the eggs until fully set and toast 2 additional split English muffins for eggwich tops.

### *Paré Pointer*
*If you want some information about a fish, just drop him a line.*

# Curry Egg Pockets

*A great breakfast to eat on the run. A convenient pocket stuffed with curried scrambled eggs, tomato, onion and cheese. Very quick and easy to prepare. If you love curry, just add a touch more.*

| | | |
|---|---|---|
| Canola oil | 1 tbsp. | 15 mL |
| Chopped tomato | 1/2 cup | 125 mL |
| Chopped green onion | 1/4 cup | 60 mL |
| Curry powder | 1 tsp. | 5 mL |
| Large eggs, fork-beaten | 6 | 6 |
| Salt, sprinkle | | |
| Pepper, sprinkle | | |
| Whole-wheat pita bread (7 inch, 18 cm, diameter), halved and opened | 2 | 2 |
| Grated medium Cheddar cheese | 1/2 cup | 125 mL |
| Chopped fresh cilantro or parsley | 1 tbsp. | 15 mL |

Heat canola oil in medium frying pan on medium. Add tomato and green onion. Cook for 2 to 3 minutes, stirring occasionally, until softened. Add curry powder. Stir. Cook for 1 minute to blend flavours.

Add eggs. Sprinkle with salt and pepper. Cook and stir until eggs are set.

Warm pita bread in microwave on high (100%) for 10 seconds. Spoon egg mixture into pita pockets. Sprinkle cheese and cilantro into pita pockets. Makes 4 pockets.

*1 pocket: 258 Calories; 14.5 g Total Fat (5.4 g Mono, 2.5 g Poly, 4.6 g Sat); 289 mg Cholesterol; 18 g Carbohydrate; 3 g Fibre; 15 g Protein; 304 mg Sodium*

 *tip* When baking or broiling food in a frying pan and the handle is not ovenproof, wrap the handle in tin foil and keep it to the front of the oven, away from the element.

# Peppered Egg Quesadilla

*Quesadillas aren't just for dinner anymore! A nutritious and delicious hand-held breakfast that's sure to please the kids.*

| | | |
|---|---|---|
| Whole-wheat flour tortillas (9 inch, 22 cm, diameter) | 2 | 2 |
| Grated jalapeño Monterey Jack cheese | 2 tbsp. | 30 mL |
| Canola oil | 1/2 tsp. | 2 mL |
| Sliced fresh white mushrooms | 1/2 cup | 125 mL |
| Chopped red pepper | 1/4 cup | 60 mL |
| Large eggs, fork-beaten | 2 | 2 |
| Chopped green onion | 2 tbsp. | 30 mL |
| Pepper | 1/8 tsp. | 0.5 mL |
| Grated jalapeño Monterey Jack cheese | 2 tbsp. | 30 mL |

Preheat oven to 400°F (205°C). Place 1 tortilla on ungreased baking sheet. Sprinkle with first amount of cheese. Set aside.

Heat canola oil in medium non-stick frying pan on medium. Add mushrooms and red pepper. Cook for about 3 minutes, stirring occasionally, until red pepper is softened.

Add eggs. Sprinkle with green onion and pepper. Reduce heat to medium-low. Cook, covered, for about 2 minutes, without stirring, until eggs are set. Slide egg mixture onto tortilla on baking sheet.

Sprinkle with second amount of cheese. Place remaining tortilla on top. Bake in oven for about 3 minutes until cheese is melted. Cut into wedges. Serves 2.

*1 serving: 274 Calories; 11.2 g Total Fat (4.2 g Mono, 1.6 g Poly, 4.5 g Sat); 199 mg Cholesterol; 37 g Carbohydrate; 4 g Fibre; 15 g Protein; 439 mg Sodium*

# Tofu Bean Dip And Crisps

*We're not trying tofu'll you, but no one's going to believe this hummus-like dip is made with tofu. With beans and a hint of salsa flavour you'll be able to aptly usher in any fiesta.*

**WHEAT POINT CRISPS**

| | | |
|---|---|---|
| Russian dressing | 2 tsp. | 10 mL |
| Ground cumin | 1/4 tsp. | 1 mL |
| Cayenne pepper, sprinkle | | |
| Whole-wheat flour tortillas<br>(9 inch, 22 cm, diameter) | 2 | 2 |

**DIP**

| | | |
|---|---|---|
| Can of white kidney beans, rinsed<br>and drained | 19 oz. | 540 mL |
| Soft tofu | 1/2 cup | 125 mL |
| Chili powder | 2 tsp. | 10 mL |
| Ground cumin | 1/2 tsp. | 2 mL |
| Garlic salt | 1/4 tsp. | 1 mL |
| Chopped tomato | 1/2 cup | 125 mL |
| Sliced green onion | 1/4 cup | 60 mL |

**Wheat Point Crisps:** Preheat oven to 425°F (220°C). Combine first 3 ingredients in small cup. Spread on tortillas. Cut each tortilla into 8 wedges. Arrange in single layer on ungreased baking sheet with sides. Bake in oven for about 5 minutes until edges are golden. Makes 16 wheat points.

**Dip:** Process first 5 ingredients in blender or food processor until smooth. Transfer to medium bowl.

Add tomato and green onion. Stir. Makes about 2 cups (500 mL) dip. Serve with Wheat Point Crisps. Serves 2.

*1 serving: 422 Calories; 8.5 g Total Fat (2.2 g Mono, 2.7 g Poly, 0.8 g Sat); 1 mg Cholesterol; 76 g Carbohydrate; 16 g Fibre; 23 g Protein; 586 mg Sodium*

Pictured on page 18.

# Red Pepper Hummus And Chips

*Roasted red peppers give hummus a sultry Mediterranean interpretation. Perfect as a dip for fresh vegetables. This hummus is also used as the spread for Greek Chicken Pockets, page 34.*

### PITA CHIPS

| | | |
|---|---|---|
| Whole-wheat pita bread (7 inch, 18 cm, diameter) | 3 | 3 |
| Olive oil | 1 tbsp. | 15 mL |

### HUMMUS

| | | |
|---|---|---|
| Can of chickpeas (garbanzo beans), rinsed and drained | 19 oz. | 540 mL |
| Roasted red peppers, drained and blotted dry | 1/2 cup | 125 mL |
| Tahini (sesame paste) | 2 tbsp. | 30 mL |
| Lemon juice | 2 tbsp. | 30 mL |
| Olive oil | 1 tbsp. | 15 mL |
| Garlic clove, minced (or 1/4 tsp., 1 mL, powder) | 1 | 1 |
| Dried oregano | 1 tsp. | 5 mL |
| Ground cumin | 1 tsp. | 5 mL |
| Salt, sprinkle (optional) | | |

**Pita Chips:** Preheat oven to 350°F (175°C). Carefully split pita bread in half horizontally to make 6 rounds. Brush first amount of olive oil on one side of each round. Stack rounds on top of each other. Cut into 8 wedges. Arrange wedges, oil side up, in single layer on 2 ungreased baking sheets with sides. Bake on separate racks in oven for about 10 minutes, switching position of baking sheets at halftime, until lightly browned. Let stand on baking sheets to cool.

**Hummus:** Meanwhile, process remaining 9 ingredients in blender or food processor until smooth. Serve with pita chips. Serves 4.

*1 serving: 453 Calories; 15.5 g Total Fat (7.4 g Mono, 4.4 g Poly, 2.0 g Sat); 0 mg Cholesterol; 65 g Carbohydrate; 10 g Fibre; 18 g Protein; 633 mg Sodium*

# Veggie Clubhouse

*With cream cheese, soft whole-wheat bread and veggies galore, this triple decker is a triple treat. To add that deli touch, secure these sandwiches with long, decorative picks.*

| | | |
|---|---|---|
| Light vegetable cream cheese | 1 tbsp. | 15 mL |
| Whole-wheat bread slice | 1 | 1 |
| Fresh spinach leaves, lightly packed | 1/4 cup | 60 mL |
| Tomato slices | 3 | 3 |
| Thin red onion slice, rings separated | 1 | 1 |
| Pepper, sprinkle | | |
| Light vegetable cream cheese | 1 tbsp. | 15 mL |
| Whole-wheat bread slice | 1 | 1 |
| English cucumber slices | 8 | 8 |
| Yellow (or red) pepper rings | 3 | 3 |
| Avocado slices (about 1/2 avocado) | 6 | 6 |
| Pepper, sprinkle | | |
| Light vegetable cream cheese | 1 tbsp. | 15 mL |
| Whole-wheat bread slice | 1 | 1 |

Spread first amount of cream cheese on 1 side of first bread slice. Layer next 3 ingredients, in order given, over cream cheese. Sprinkle with pepper.

Spread second amount of cream cheese on both sides of second bread slice. Place on top of onion. Layer next 3 ingredients, in order given, over cream cheese. Sprinkle with pepper.

Spread third amount of cream cheese on 1 side of third bread slice. Place, cream cheese-side down, on top of sandwich. Cut sandwich diagonally into 4 small triangles. Makes 1 sandwich.

*1 sandwich: 452 Calories; 25.6 g Total Fat (1.4 g Mono, 1.0 g Poly, 6.6 g Sat); 30 mg Cholesterol; 54 g Carbohydrate; 10 g Fibre; 15 g Protein; 698 mg Sodium*

Pictured on page 35.

# Turkey Pear Sandwich

*A gourmet sandwich shop couldn't do any better! This tasty treat is similar to a clubhouse but uses pear instead of bacon.*

| | | |
|---|---|---|
| Light mayonnaise | 4 tsp. | 20 mL |
| Whole-wheat bread slices | 4 | 4 |
| Chopped pecans, toasted (see Tip, page 14) | 1 tbsp. | 15 mL |
| Fresh small pear, sliced (see Note) | 1 | 1 |
| Lean deli smoked turkey breast slices (about 4 oz., 113 g) | 4 | 4 |
| Salt, sprinkle | | |
| Pepper, sprinkle | | |
| Thin slices of light Havarti cheese | 2 | 2 |
| Small Roma (plum) tomato, thinly sliced | 1 | 1 |
| Butter lettuce leaves | 6 – 8 | 6 – 8 |

Spread mayonnaise on bread slices. Sprinkle pecans over mayonnaise on 2 bread slices.

Arrange pear slices over pecans.

Loosely roll turkey slices and place over pear. Sprinkle with salt and pepper.

Arrange next 3 ingredients, in order given, over turkey. Top with remaining bread slices, mayonnaise-side down. Cut sandwiches in half. Makes 2 sandwiches.

*1 sandwich: 436 Calories; 19.9 g Total Fat (2.5 g Mono, 1.5 g Poly, 7.4 g Sat); 64 mg Cholesterol; 42 g Carbohydrate; 7 g Fibre; 27 g Protein; 1065 mg Sodium*

**Note:** If not eating sandwich right away, dip pear in acidulated water (about 1 tsp., 5 mL, lemon juice and 1/2 cup, 125 mL, water) and drain on paper towel before adding to sandwich.

# Modern Caesar Pitas

*Don't get your toga in a tangle, this update on an old favourite is sure to please. What makes these pitas so pleasingly different? The added flavours of tahini and walnuts. All hail Caesar!*

| | | |
|---|---|---|
| Chopped or torn romaine lettuce, lightly packed | 3 cups | 750 mL |
| Diced cooked chicken | 1 cup | 250 mL |
| Chopped walnuts | 1/4 cup | 60 mL |
| GARLIC SESAME DRESSING | | |
| Olive oil | 1 tbsp. | 15 mL |
| Lemon juice | 1 tbsp. | 15 mL |
| White wine vinegar | 1 tbsp. | 15 mL |
| Tahini (sesame paste) | 1 tbsp. | 15 mL |
| Anchovy paste (optional) | 1/4 tsp. | 1 mL |
| Garlic clove, minced (or 1/4 tsp., 1 mL, powder) | 1 | 1 |
| Pepper | 1/8 tsp. | 0.5 mL |
| Whole-wheat pita bread (7 inch, 18 cm, diameter), halved and opened | 2 | 2 |

Put first 3 ingredients into medium bowl.

**Garlic Sesame Dressing:** Beat first 7 ingredients with fork in small cup. Makes about 1/4 cup (60 mL) dressing. Pour over lettuce mixture. Toss well.

Spoon lettuce mixture into pita pockets. Makes 4 pitas.

*1 pita: 243 Calories; 13.4 g Total Fat (4.9 g Mono, 5.6 g Poly, 2.0 g Sat); 26 mg Cholesterol; 19 g Carbohydrate; 4 g Fibre; 14 g Protein; 182 mg Sodium*

## *Paré Pointer*

*Cross a snowman and a vampire and you'll get frostbite.*

# Asian Chicken Wraps

*An Asian-influenced wrap with a great coleslaw crunch similar to that of bean sprouts. Don't shy away from adding your own special touches, such as sliced mushrooms, shredded carrot or chopped pepper.*

| | | |
|---|---|---|
| Coleslaw mix | 1 1/2 cups | 375 mL |
| Chopped cooked chicken | 1 cup | 250 mL |
| Chopped green onion | 1/4 cup | 60 mL |
| Sesame seeds, toasted (see Tip, page 14) | 1 tbsp. | 15 mL |
| **HONEY SOY DRESSING** | | |
| Rice vinegar | 1 tbsp. | 15 mL |
| Liquid honey | 1 tbsp. | 15 mL |
| Olive oil | 2 tsp. | 10 mL |
| Low-sodium soy sauce | 2 tsp. | 10 mL |
| Cayenne pepper, just a pinch | | |
| Green leaf lettuce leaves, centre ribs removed (see Tip, page 110) | 4 | 4 |
| Whole-wheat flour tortillas (9 inch, 22 cm, diameter) | 2 | 2 |

Combine first 4 ingredients in medium bowl.

**Honey Soy Dressing:** Combine first 5 ingredients in small cup. Makes about 3 tbsp. (50 mL) dressing. Drizzle over coleslaw mixture. Toss well.

Place 2 lettuce leaves on each tortilla. Spoon coleslaw mixture over lettuce down centre of tortillas. Fold bottom ends of tortillas over filling. Fold in sides, leaving top ends open. Makes 2 wraps.

*1 wrap: 366 Calories; 12.2 g Total Fat (6.0 g Mono, 2.8 g Poly, 2.3 g Sat); 53 mg Cholesterol; 49 g Carbohydrate; 5 g Fibre; 24 g Protein; 533 mg Sodium*

# Chipotle Lime Dip

*Use this multipurpose dip whenever you want some southwestern zing.*
*Serve with veggies or the chips from Red Pepper Hummus And Chips,*
*page 25. Also try as a spread on Polenta Vegetable Stacks, page 109.*

| | | |
|---|---|---|
| Light sour cream | 1/2 cup | 125 mL |
| Light mayonnaise | 1/2 cup | 125 mL |
| Lime juice | 1/4 cup | 60 mL |
| Chopped fresh cilantro or parsley | 1/4 cup | 60 mL |
| Minced chipotle peppers in adobo sauce (see Tip, page 76) | 1 tbsp. | 15 mL |
| Grated lime zest | 2 tsp. | 10 mL |

Combine all 6 ingredients in small bowl. Makes about 1 1/3 cups (325 mL).

*1/4 cup (60 mL): 116 Calories; 9.7 g Total Fat (trace Mono, trace Poly, 2.3 g Sat); 16 mg Cholesterol;*
*5 g Carbohydrate; trace Fibre; 2 g Protein; 204 mg Sodium*

# Cottage Fruit Salad

*Just call it fruit salad deluxe! Serve with rye toast or stuff into a lettuce-lined*
*pita pocket to make a tasty fruit sandwich.*

| | | |
|---|---|---|
| 1% cottage cheese | 1 1/2 cups | 375 mL |
| Small tart apple (such as Granny Smith), diced | 1 | 1 |
| Chopped celery | 1/4 cup | 60 mL |
| Dried cranberries | 1/4 cup | 60 mL |
| Raisins | 2 tbsp. | 30 mL |
| Pecan pieces, toasted (see Tip, page 14) | 2 tbsp. | 30 mL |
| Walnut pieces, toasted (see Tip, page 14) | 2 tbsp. | 30 mL |
| Liquid honey | 1 tbsp. | 15 mL |
| Ground cinnamon | 1/2 tsp. | 2 mL |

Combine all 9 ingredients in medium bowl. Mix well. Makes about
2 1/2 cups (625 mL).

*1 cup (250 mL): 301 Calories; 10.0 g Total Fat (3.4 g Mono, 4.3 g Poly, 1.7 g Sat); 6 mg Cholesterol;*
*37 g Carbohydrate; 4 g Fibre; 19 g Protein; 580 mg Sodium*

# Ham And Chicken Stack

*One giant sandwich stacked with enough ham, chicken and vegetables to serve six! For easier cutting, secure sandwich in six places with long picks before cutting into wedges. Looks as colossal as it tastes!*

| | | |
|---|---|---|
| Herb focaccia bread (10 inch, 25 cm, diameter) | 1 | 1 |
| Olive oil | 2 tsp. | 10 mL |
| **SWEET MUSTARD MAYO** | | |
| Dijon mustard | 3 tbsp. | 50 mL |
| Liquid honey | 2 tbsp. | 30 mL |
| Light mayonnaise | 1 tbsp. | 15 mL |
| Finely chopped fresh rosemary (or 1/8 tsp., 0.5 mL, dried, crushed) | 1/2 tsp. | 2 mL |
| **FILLING** | | |
| Romaine lettuce leaves | 4 | 4 |
| Thin slices of yellow pepper | 8 | 8 |
| Thin slices of tomato | 6 | 6 |
| No-fat deli ham slices (about 4 1/2 oz., 125 g) | 5 | 5 |
| Sliced cooked chicken breast | 1 1/4 cups | 300 mL |

Preheat broiler. Cut focaccia bread in half horizontally. Brush cut sides with olive oil. Place, cut side up, on ungreased baking sheet. Broil on top rack in oven for about 2 minutes until golden. Transfer to cutting surface.

**Sweet Mustard Mayo:** Combine all 4 ingredients in small bowl. Makes about 6 tbsp. (100 mL) mayo. Spread on toasted focaccia.

**Filling:** Place lettuce leaves on bottom half of focaccia. Layer remaining 4 ingredients, in order given, over lettuce. Cover with top half of focaccia. Cut into 6 wedges. Serves 6.

*1 wedge: 241 Calories; 5.2 g Total Fat (1.6 g Mono, 0.4 g Poly, 0.7 g Sat); 28 mg Cholesterol; 35 g Carbohydrate; 1 g Fibre; 14 g Protein; 596 mg Sodium*

Pictured on page 35.

# Tuna Mango Wraps

*This fresh, light sandwich alternative is a unique diversion from everyday luncheon fare. Line the wrap with spinach first to keep it from getting soggy. Try with fresh mango when it's in season.*

| | | |
|---|---|---|
| Frozen (or fresh) mango pieces, thawed, drained and chopped | 1 cup | 250 mL |
| Can of flaked white tuna in water, drained | 6 oz. | 170 g |
| Light mayonnaise | 2 tbsp. | 30 mL |
| Chopped green onion | 1 tbsp. | 15 mL |
| Low-sodium soy sauce | 1 1/2 tsp. | 7 mL |
| Lime juice | 1 tsp. | 5 mL |
| Fresh spinach leaves, lightly packed | 1/2 cup | 125 mL |
| Whole-wheat flour tortillas (9 inch, 22 cm, diameter) | 2 | 2 |

Combine first 6 ingredients in small bowl.

Arrange spinach along centre of tortillas. Spoon tuna mixture over spinach. Fold bottom ends of tortillas over filling. Fold in sides, leaving top ends open. Makes 2 wraps.

*1 wrap: 347 Calories; 8.5 g Total Fat (0.9 g Mono, 1.3 g Poly, 1.6 g Sat); 41 mg Cholesterol; 51 g Carbohydrate; 5 g Fibre; 26 g Protein; 601 mg Sodium*

# Summer Cucumber Sandwiches

*For those who like to crunch, this sandwich is for you. A garden-inspired spread that tastes great on all your favourite breads.*

| | | |
|---|---|---|
| Light vegetable cream cheese | 1/4 cup | 60 mL |
| Minced radish | 1/4 cup | 60 mL |
| Light rye bread slices | 4 | 4 |
| Raw sunflower seeds | 1 tsp. | 5 mL |
| Salt, sprinkle | | |
| Pepper, sprinkle | | |
| Slices of English cucumber (with peel) | 12 | 12 |
| Alfalfa sprouts, lightly packed | 1/3 cup | 75 mL |

*(continued on next page)*

Mix cream cheese and radish in small bowl. Spread mixture on 4 bread slices.

Sprinkle next 3 ingredients over cream cheese mixture on 2 bread slices.

Arrange cucumber slices and alfalfa sprouts over sunflower seeds. Top with remaining bread slices, cream cheese-side down. Cut sandwiches in half. Serves 2.

*1 serving: 242 Calories; 7.2 g Total Fat (0.9 g Mono, 0.6 g Poly, 3.6 g Sat); 20 mg Cholesterol; 35 g Carbohydrate; 4 g Fibre; 8 g Protein; 591 mg Sodium*

**Variation:** Use goat (chèvre) cheese instead of cream cheese.

---

# Tomato Bagel Melts

*This quick and hearty sandwich is made special with the clever addition of Asiago cheese and olives. For a milder flavour, try the Bocconcini Salad Melts variation.*

| | | |
|---|---|---|
| Whole-wheat bagels, split | 4 | 4 |
| Chopped fresh basil | 1/4 cup | 60 mL |
| Sliced black olives | 1/4 cup | 60 mL |
| Thinly sliced medium tomatoes | 2 | 2 |
| Pepper | 1/4 tsp. | 1 mL |
| Grated Asiago cheese | 1/2 cup | 125 mL |

Preheat broiler. Arrange bagel halves, cut side up, on ungreased baking sheet. Broil on top rack in oven for about 2 minutes until lightly golden and toasted. Cover top halves of bagels to keep warm.

Arrange next 3 ingredients on bottom halves of bagels. Sprinkle with pepper.

Sprinkle with cheese. Broil on top rack in oven for 2 to 3 minutes until cheese is melted. Top with remaining bagel halves. Let stand for 1 minute. Press down lightly to squeeze cheese between layers. Cut bagels in half. Makes 4 sandwiches.

*1 sandwich: 493 Calories; 16.4 g Total Fat (1.0 g Mono, 0.8 g Poly, 8.0 g Sat); 38 mg Cholesterol; 69 g Carbohydrate; 13 g Fibre; 22 g Protein; 1097 mg Sodium*

**BOCCONCINI SALAD MELTS:** Use slices of bocconcini cheese instead of Asiago and sprinkle with a bit more pepper.

# Greek Chicken Pockets

*You don't have to be Zorba to enjoy these tzatziki-inspired (pronounced dzah-DZEE-kee) pita pockets. Red Pepper Hummus, page 25, is used as a spread for this recipe but you may want to substitute with a family favourite spread instead.*

| | | |
|---|---|---|
| Red Pepper Hummus, page 25 | 1/4 cup | 60 mL |
| Whole-wheat pita bread (7 inch, 18 cm, diameter), halved and opened | 2 | 2 |
| Chopped cooked chicken | 1 cup | 250 mL |
| Thinly sliced red pepper | 1/2 cup | 125 mL |
| Plain yogurt | 1/3 cup | 75 mL |
| Chopped tomato | 1/4 cup | 60 mL |
| Chopped pitted kalamata (or black) olives | 1/4 cup | 60 mL |
| Finely chopped English cucumber | 1/4 cup | 60 mL |
| Chopped red onion | 2 tbsp. | 30 mL |
| Chopped fresh oregano (or 3/4 tsp., 4 mL, dried) | 1 tbsp. | 15 mL |
| Pepper | 1/4 tsp. | 1 mL |

Spread hummus inside pita pockets.

Combine remaining 9 ingredients in medium bowl. Spoon into pita pockets. Makes 4 pockets.

*1 pocket: 193 Calories; 5.5 g Total Fat (2.2 g Mono, 1.3 g Poly, 1.3 g Sat); 29 mg Cholesterol; 23 g Carbohydrate; 4 g Fibre; 14 g Protein; 318 mg Sodium*

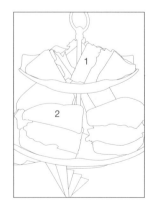

1. Veggie Clubhouse, page 26
2. Ham And Chicken Stack, page 31

Props courtesy of: Cherison Enterprises Inc.

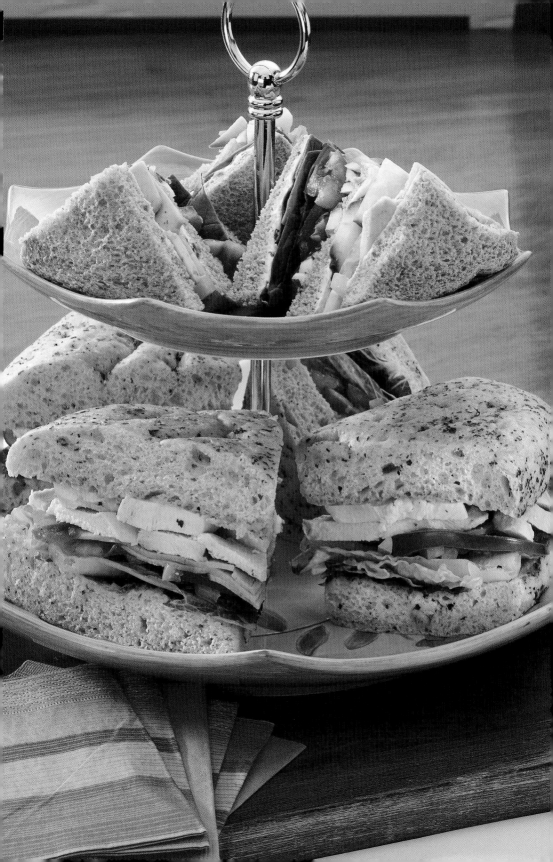

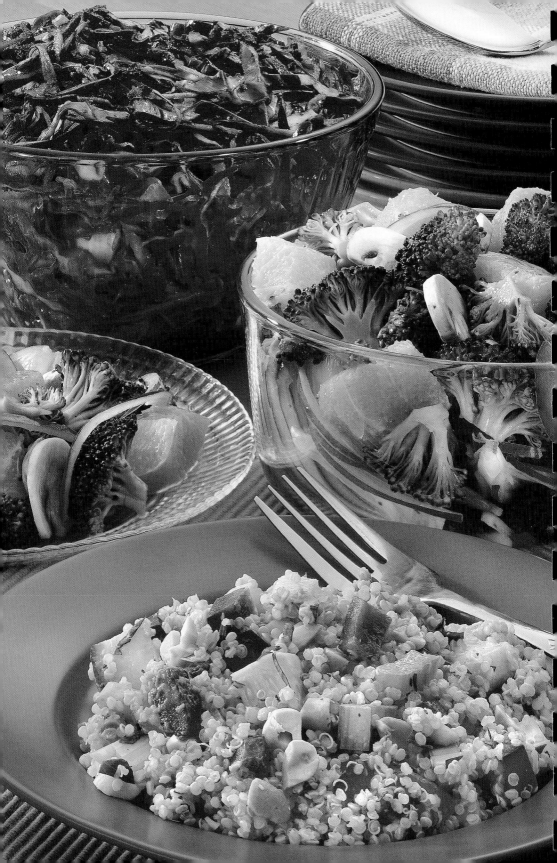

# Apple Carrot Slaw

*I'm sure you slaw this coming—an apple coleslaw with a spicy heat. The addition of figs adds a pleasant, chewy sweetness. Best served immediately.*

| | | |
|---|---|---|
| Grated carrot | 2 cups | 500 mL |
| Medium tart apples (such as Granny Smith), peeled and grated | 2 | 2 |
| Chopped dried figs | 1/4 cup | 60 mL |
| Chopped fresh parsley | 1/4 cup | 60 mL |
| Chopped pecans | 1/4 cup | 60 mL |
| **SPICY ORANGE DRESSING** | | |
| Orange juice | 1/2 cup | 125 mL |
| Flax (or olive) oil | 2 tbsp. | 30 mL |
| Granulated sugar | 2 tsp. | 10 mL |
| Ground cinnamon | 1/4 tsp. | 1 mL |
| Ground cumin | 1/4 tsp. | 1 mL |
| Cayenne pepper | 1/8 tsp. | 0.5 mL |

Combine first 5 ingredients in medium bowl. Toss.

**Spicy Orange Dressing:** Whisk all 6 ingredients in small bowl until combined. Makes about 2/3 cup (150 mL) dressing. Drizzle over salad. Toss well. Serves 4.

*1 serving: 220 Calories; 12.6 g Total Fat (4.4 g Mono, 6.3 g Poly, 1.2 g Sat); 0 mg Cholesterol; 28 g Carbohydrate; 5 g Fibre; 2 g Protein; 42 mg Sodium*

Pictured on page 71 and on back cover.

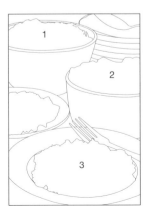

1. Balsamic Slaw, page 39
2. Broccoli Orange Salad, page 41
3. Nutty Quinoa Salad, page 38

Props courtesy of: Danesco Inc.
Casa Bugatti

# Nutty Quinoa Salad

*You'll be nutty about this vegetable-packed salad with a zippy dressing. Quinoa (pronounced KEEN–wah) is a tasty alternative in salads that usually use couscous or bulgur. Find it in the bulk or health food sections of most grocery stores.*

**SALAD**

| | | |
|---|---|---|
| Water | 1 1/2 cups | 375 mL |
| Quinoa, rinsed and drained | 3/4 cup | 175 mL |
| Chopped red pepper | 1/2 cup | 125 mL |
| Chopped celery | 1/2 cup | 125 mL |
| Diced English cucumber | 1/2 cup | 125 mL |
| Finely chopped green onion | 1/4 cup | 60 mL |
| Chopped fresh cilantro or parsley | 2 tbsp. | 30 mL |
| Salt, sprinkle | | |

**NUTTY LIME DRESSING**

| | | |
|---|---|---|
| Chunky peanut butter | 3 tbsp. | 50 mL |
| Lime juice | 2 tbsp. | 30 mL |
| Rice vinegar | 2 tbsp. | 30 mL |
| Low-sodium soy sauce | 2 tsp. | 10 mL |
| Garlic clove, minced | 1 | 1 |
| (or 1/4 tsp., 1 mL, powder) | | |
| Finely grated ginger root | 2 tsp. | 10 mL |
| (or 1/2 tsp., 2 mL, ground ginger) | | |
| Cayenne pepper | 1/8 tsp. | 0.5 mL |

**TOPPING**

| | | |
|---|---|---|
| Chopped salted peanuts | 1/3 cup | 75 mL |

**Salad:** Combine water and quinoa in medium saucepan. Bring to a boil. Reduce heat to medium-low. Simmer, covered, for about 15 minutes until water is absorbed. Transfer to baking sheet with sides. Spread in thin layer. Chill for 5 to 10 minutes until cool.

Meanwhile, combine next 6 ingredients in medium bowl.

**Nutty Lime Dressing:** Whisk all 7 ingredients in small bowl until combined. Makes about 1/2 cup (125 mL) dressing. Drizzle over salad. Add quinoa. Mix well.

**Topping:** Sprinkle with peanuts. Serves 4.

*(continued on next page)*

*1 serving: 273 Calories; 13.7 g Total Fat (6.3 g Mono, 4.4 g Poly, 2.0 g Sat); 0 mg Cholesterol; 31 g Carbohydrate; 5 g Fibre; 10 g Protein; 256 mg Sodium*

Pictured on page 36.

**TAHINI LIME DRESSING:** Use the same amount of tahini (sesame paste) instead of peanut butter.

# Balsamic Slaw

*Slaw down and take the time to enjoy this tangy treat. The unique shades of this purple and orange salad will add colour to any entree.*

| | | |
|---|---|---|
| Shredded red cabbage, lightly packed | 4 cups | 1 L |
| Can of whole baby beets, drained, grated (see Tip, page 47) | 14 oz. | 398 mL |
| Grated carrot | 1 1/2 cups | 375 mL |
| Thinly sliced red onion | 1/4 cup | 60 mL |
| BALSAMIC DRESSING | | |
| Balsamic vinegar | 1/4 cup | 60 mL |
| Olive oil | 1/4 cup | 60 mL |
| Chili sauce | 2 tbsp. | 30 mL |
| Lemon juice | 1 tbsp. | 15 mL |
| Granulated sugar | 1 tbsp. | 15 mL |
| Salt | 1/8 tsp. | 0.5 mL |
| Pepper | 1/8 tsp. | 0.5 mL |

Put first 4 ingredients into large bowl.

**Balsamic Dressing:** Whisk all 7 ingredients in small bowl until combined. Makes about 3/4 cup (175 mL) dressing. Drizzle over salad. Toss well. Serves 6.

*1 serving: 150 Calories; 9.4 g Total Fat (6.7 g Mono, 0.9 g Poly, 1.3 g Sat); 0 mg Cholesterol; 16 g Carbohydrate; 3 g Fibre; 2 g Protein; 356 mg Sodium*

Pictured on page 36.

 It's time to get keen on quinoa. It cooks quickly and contains all of the 9 essential amino acids your body needs to build new cells. Before cooking, remember to give it a quick rinse to remove any residue that may impart a bitter taste.

# Portobellos And Greens

*Fresh and summery—both in flavour and appearance. Make this salad a meal by bulking it up with cooked chickpeas or other beans. Grilling the asparagus will enhance its natural flavour.*

| | | |
|---|---|---|
| Portobello mushrooms, stems removed | 2 | 2 |
| Fresh asparagus, trimmed of tough ends | 1/2 lb. | 225 g |
| Olive oil | 1 1/2 tbsp. | 25 mL |
| Salt, sprinkle | | |
| Pepper, sprinkle | | |
| **SUN-DRIED TOMATO DRESSING** | | |
| Red wine vinegar | 2 tbsp. | 30 mL |
| Sun-dried tomato pesto | 1 tbsp. | 15 mL |
| Olive oil | 1 tbsp. | 15 mL |
| Balsamic vinegar | 1 tbsp. | 15 mL |
| Chopped or torn romaine lettuce, lightly packed | 6 cups | 1.5 L |
| Crumbled light feta cheese | 1/2 cup | 125 mL |

Preheat gas barbecue to medium (see Note). Arrange mushrooms and asparagus on large plate. Brush with olive oil. Sprinkle with salt and pepper. Grill mushrooms for about 5 minutes per side until tender. Grill asparagus for 3 to 4 minutes, turning several times, until tender-crisp. Cut mushrooms into bite-size slices. Cut asparagus crosswise into 3 pieces each. Transfer to extra-large bowl. Set aside.

**Sun-Dried Tomato Dressing:** Whisk all 4 ingredients in small bowl until combined. Makes about 1/3 cup (75 mL) dressing.

Add lettuce and feta cheese to mushroom mixture. Drizzle with dressing. Toss well. Serves 4.

*1 serving: 171 Calories; 12.5 g Total Fat (7.2 g Mono, 1.0 g Poly, 2.9 g Sat); 8 mg Cholesterol; 9 g Carbohydrate; 3 g Fibre; 8 g Protein; 305 mg Sodium*

Pictured on page 125.

**Note:** Too cold to barbecue? Mushrooms and asparagus can be placed on a greased broiling pan and broiled on top rack in oven. Broil mushrooms for about 5 minutes per side until tender. Broil asparagus for 3 to 4 minutes, turning several times, until tender-crisp.

# Broccoli Orange Salad

*The perfect busy-day salad! Easy to make ahead of time because ingredients will stay fresh without dressing for an hour or more. Toss with dressing just before serving.*

**TANGY ORANGE DRESSING**

| | | |
|---|---|---|
| Frozen concentrated orange juice, thawed | 1/4 cup | 60 mL |
| Sesame (or canola) oil | 2 tbsp. | 30 mL |
| Rice vinegar | 2 tbsp. | 30 mL |
| Dry mustard | 1/2 tsp. | 2 mL |
| Salt | 1/4 tsp. | 1 mL |

**SALAD**

| | | |
|---|---|---|
| Broccoli florets | 4 cups | 1 L |
| Water | 1 tbsp. | 15 mL |
| Medium oranges, peeled and cut into 1 inch (2.5 cm) pieces | 3 | 3 |
| Sliced fresh white mushrooms | 1 cup | 250 mL |
| Sliced red onion | 1/4 cup | 60 mL |

**Tangy Orange Dressing:** Whisk first 5 ingredients in small bowl until combined. Makes about 1/2 cup (125 mL) dressing. Set aside.

**Salad:** Arrange broccoli on large microwave-safe plate. Sprinkle with water. Microwave, covered, on high (100%) for about 2 minutes until broccoli begins to soften and turn bright green. Transfer to large bowl.

Add remaining 3 ingredients. Drizzle with dressing. Toss. Serves 4.

*1 serving: 170 Calories; 7.1 g Total Fat (2.7 g Mono, 2.9 g Poly, 1.0 g Sat); 0 mg Cholesterol; 28 g Carbohydrate; 8 g Fibre; 4 g Protein; 139 mg Sodium*

Pictured on page 36.

*fyi*　Instead of an orange, why not go for a mango? Mango is rich in Vitamin C, which is very important in maintaining a healthy immune system. It is also high in dietary fibre and low in calories. When selecting a mango, choose one with a firm, unblemished skin and a sweet, tropical scent at the stem end. A ripe mango will also have a little bit of give when you squeeze it gently.

# Cool Beets And Beans

*Up your dinner's cool factor with this colourful, multi-textured salad tossed with a refreshing orange dressing. Serve with whole-grain bread.*

| | | |
|---|---|---|
| Olive (or canola) oil | 3 tbsp. | 50 mL |
| Frozen concentrated orange juice, thawed | 2 tbsp. | 30 mL |
| Red wine vinegar | 1 tbsp. | 15 mL |
| Chopped fresh dill (or 1/2 tsp., 2 mL, dried) | 2 tsp. | 10 mL |
| Salt | 1/8 tsp. | 0.5 mL |
| Pepper | 1/8 tsp. | 0.5 mL |
| Chopped or torn romaine lettuce, lightly packed | 3 cups | 750 mL |
| Can of chickpeas (garbanzo beans), rinsed and drained | 19 oz. | 540 mL |
| Can of whole baby beets, drained and chopped (see Tip, page 47) | 14 oz. | 398 mL |
| Grated carrot | 1 cup | 250 mL |
| Salted, roasted shelled pumpkin seeds | 1/4 cup | 60 mL |

Whisk first 6 ingredients in large bowl until combined.

Add remaining 5 ingredients. Toss well. Serves 4.

*1 serving: 448 Calories; 20.0 g Total Fat (10.2 g Mono, 5.3 g Poly, 2.9 g Sat); 0 mg Cholesterol; 53 g Carbohydrate; 10 g Fibre; 19 g Protein; 684 mg Sodium*

# Lemony White Bean Salad

*Crisp romaine all dressed up with juicy tomatoes and soft beans. Use spinach instead of romaine for an extra iron boost.*

| | | |
|---|---|---|
| Can of white kidney beans, rinsed and drained | 19 oz. | 540 mL |
| Ranch dressing | 1/4 cup | 60 mL |
| Lemon juice | 1 tbsp. | 15 mL |
| Grated lemon zest | 1 tsp. | 5 mL |
| Chopped or torn romaine lettuce, lightly packed | 8 cups | 2 L |
| Grape tomatoes, halved | 2/3 cup | 150 mL |
| Thinly sliced red onion | 1/4 cup | 60 mL |

*(continued on next page)*

Salads

Combine first 4 ingredients in large bowl.

Add remaining 3 ingredients. Toss. Serves 6.

*1 serving: 136 Calories; 6.1 g Total Fat (trace Mono, 0.1 g Poly, 0.8 g Sat); 3 mg Cholesterol; 16 g Carbohydrate; 5 g Fibre; 6 g Protein; 132 mg Sodium*

---

# Summer Salad

*"In the summertime when the weather is fine…" use fresh raspberries, but when the weather is less than fine frozen will do, too. The goat cheese and raspberries are a heavenly combination.*

| | | |
|---|---|---|
| Spring mix lettuce, lightly packed | 6 cups | 1.5 L |
| Fresh (or frozen) raspberries | 1 cup | 250 mL |
| Goat (chèvre) cheese, crumbled (see Tip, below) | 2 1/2 oz. | 70 g |
| Sliced natural almonds, toasted (see Tip, page 14) | 1/4 cup | 60 mL |
| **SWEET VINAIGRETTE** | | |
| Olive (or canola) oil | 3 tbsp. | 50 mL |
| White vinegar | 2 tbsp. | 30 mL |
| Granulated sugar | 2 tbsp. | 30 mL |
| Dry mustard | 1 tsp. | 5 mL |
| Salt, sprinkle | | |
| Pepper, sprinkle | | |

Put first 4 ingredients into large bowl.

**Sweet Vinaigrette:** Whisk all 6 ingredients in small bowl until combined. Makes about 1/3 cup (75 mL) dressing. Drizzle over salad. Toss. Serves 4.

*1 serving: 230 Calories; 18.1 g Total Fat (10.2 g Mono, 1.8 g Poly, 4.6 g Sat); 10 mg Cholesterol; 12 g Carbohydrate; 3 g Fibre; 6 g Protein; 83 mg Sodium*

Pictured on page 143.

 To grate or crumble soft cheese easily, place in the freezer for 15 to 20 minutes until very firm.

# Creamy Pasta Salad

*Not your ordinary pasta salad! Packed with personality, this twist on a sometimes lacklustre staple is an excellent way to sneak some tofu into your diet. See the variation below for a spicier dressing that is also great as a vegetable dip.*

| | | |
|---|---|---|
| Whole-wheat rotini | 2 cups | 500 mL |
| **CREAMY TOFU DRESSING** | | |
| Soft tofu | 1/2 cup | 125 mL |
| Italian seasoning | 1 tsp. | 5 mL |
| Dijon mustard | 1 tbsp. | 15 mL |
| Lemon juice | 1 tbsp. | 15 mL |
| Garlic cloves, minced | 1 – 2 | 1 – 2 |
| Pepper | 1/4 tsp. | 1 mL |
| Can of artichoke hearts, drained and chopped | 14 oz. | 398 mL |
| Chopped red pepper | 3/4 cup | 175 mL |
| Chopped green onion | 1/4 cup | 60 mL |
| Pine nuts | 1/4 cup | 60 mL |

Cook pasta in boiling salted water in large uncovered saucepan or Dutch oven for about 10 minutes until tender but firm. Drain. Rinse with cold water. Drain. Transfer to large bowl.

**Creamy Tofu Dressing:** Meanwhile, combine all 6 ingredients in small bowl. Process with hand blender until smooth. Makes about 3/4 cup (175 mL) dressing.

Add remaining 4 ingredients to pasta. Add dressing. Toss well. Serves 4.

*1 serving: 279 Calories; 7.2 g Total Fat (2.3 g Mono, 3.1 g Poly, 1.1 g Sat); 0 mg Cholesterol; 46 g Carbohydrate; 11 g Fibre; 15 g Protein; 209 mg Sodium*

Pictured on page 71 and on back cover.

**CREAMY CHIPOTLE DRESSING:** Add 1 minced chipotle pepper (see Tip, page 76) to Creamy Tofu Dressing.

# Bulgur Chicken Salad

*The perfect blend of fresh and tangy, this little taste treat does double duty—
serve it warm or chilled.*

| | | |
|---|---|---|
| Prepared chicken broth | 2 cups | 500 mL |
| Frozen cut green beans | 2 cups | 500 mL |
| Bulgur, fine grind | 1 cup | 250 mL |
| Chopped cooked chicken | 3 cups | 750 mL |
| Chopped red onion | 1/2 cup | 125 mL |
| Dried cranberries (or raisins) | 1/2 cup | 125 mL |
| Chopped fresh mint (or basil) | 1/3 cup | 75 mL |
| Olive oil | 1/4 cup | 60 mL |
| Plain yogurt | 3 tbsp. | 50 mL |
| Lemon juice | 3 tbsp. | 50 mL |
| Salt | 1/2 tsp. | 2 mL |
| Pepper | 1/4 tsp. | 1 mL |
| Red leaf lettuce leaves | 12 | 12 |

Measure broth and green beans into medium saucepan. Bring to a boil.
Remove from heat.

Add bulgur. Stir. Cover. Let stand for about 20 minutes until broth
is absorbed.

Add next 4 ingredients. Stir.

Whisk next 5 ingredients in small bowl until combined. Pour over chicken
mixture. Toss.

Arrange lettuce leaves on 6 salad plates. Spoon chicken mixture over
lettuce. Serves 6.

*1 serving: 355 Calories; 14.9 g Total Fat (8.8 g Mono, 2.1 g Poly, 2.9 g Sat); 54 mg Cholesterol;
32 g Carbohydrate; 5 g Fibre; 23 g Protein; 534 mg Sodium*

 Instead of adding cooked chicken or beef to a salad, add a juicy
grilled portobello mushroom instead. It will give you a satisfying
meaty texture without the meat!

# Curried Tofu Spinach Salad

*It's yellow—but it's sure not mellow! Bright yellow cubes of curried tofu are
sure to stand out in this uniquely spicy and sweet flavour combination.*

| | | |
|---|---|---|
| Curry powder | 1 tbsp. | 15 mL |
| Cornstarch | 1 tbsp. | 15 mL |
| Salt | 1 tsp. | 5 mL |
| Package of firm tofu, cut into 1/2 inch (12 mm) cubes | 12 1/4 oz. | 350 g |
| Olive oil | 1 tbsp. | 15 mL |
| MANGO DRESSING | | |
| Mango chutney, larger pieces chopped | 1/4 cup | 60 mL |
| Lime juice | 2 tbsp. | 30 mL |
| Olive oil | 1 tbsp. | 15 mL |
| Fresh spinach leaves, lightly packed | 5 cups | 1.25 L |
| Sliced natural almonds, toasted (see Tip, page 14) | 2 tbsp. | 30 mL |

Combine first 3 ingredients in shallow bowl.

Pat tofu dry with paper towel. Add to curry mixture. Toss until coated.

Heat olive oil in medium frying pan on medium. Add tofu. Cook for about
8 minutes, stirring occasionally, until golden and crisp on outside.

**Mango Dressing:** Meanwhile, whisk first 3 ingredients in large bowl until
combined. Makes about 1/2 cup (125 mL) dressing.

Add spinach. Toss well. Arrange on 4 salad plates.

Sprinkle with almonds and tofu. Serves 4.

*1 serving: 188 Calories; 11.2 g Total Fat (6.5 g Mono, 2.4 g Poly, 1.5 g Sat); 0 mg Cholesterol;
15 g Carbohydrate; 3 g Fibre; 9 g Protein; 676 mg Sodium*

# Baby Potato Sage Toss

*Earthy sage, sweet honey and tangy Dijon coat roasted potatoes and crisp sugar snap peas in this splendid summertime salad that perfectly complements grilled meats.*

| | | |
|---|---|---|
| Baby red potatoes, quartered | 1 lb. | 454 g |
| Chopped fresh sage | 2 tbsp. | 30 mL |
| Olive oil | 1 tbsp. | 15 mL |
| **HONEY DIJON DRESSING** | | |
| Olive oil | 2 tbsp. | 30 mL |
| White vinegar | 2 tbsp. | 30 mL |
| Liquid honey | 2 tsp. | 10 mL |
| Dijon (or prepared) mustard | 1/2 tsp. | 2 mL |
| Chopped or torn green leaf lettuce, lightly packed | 4 cups | 1 L |
| Sugar snap peas, trimmed and halved | 1 cup | 250 mL |
| Chopped green onion | 1/3 cup | 75 mL |

Preheat oven to 400°F (205°C). Combine first 3 ingredients in large bowl. Toss well. Spread in single layer in ungreased 9 × 13 inch (22 × 33 cm) baking dish. Bake in oven for about 15 minutes until tender.

**Honey Dijon Dressing:** Meanwhile, whisk all 4 ingredients in small bowl until combined. Makes about 1/4 cup (75 mL) dressing.

Combine remaining 3 ingredients in large bowl. Add potatoes and dressing. Toss well. Serves 4.

*1 serving: 231 Calories; 10.5 g Total Fat (7.5 g Mono, 1.0 g Poly, 1.4 g Sat); 0 mg Cholesterol; 30 g Carbohydrate; 4 g Fibre; 4 g Protein; 28 mg Sodium*

Pictured on page 54.

 *tip* Don't get caught red-handed! Wear rubber gloves when handling beets.

# Grilled Beef Salad

*Daikon, a juicy, long, white Asian radish, has a peppery flavour and crunch that is well-matched with the spicy beef and sesame dressing in this exotic taste treat.*

| | | |
|---|---|---|
| Beef strip loin steak | 3/4 lb. | 340 g |
| Chili paste (sambal oelek) | 2 tsp. | 10 mL |
| **SESAME LIME DRESSING** | | |
| Lime juice | 1/4 cup | 60 mL |
| Sesame oil | 2 tbsp. | 30 mL |
| Low-sodium soy sauce | 2 tbsp. | 30 mL |
| Brown sugar, packed | 2 tbsp. | 30 mL |
| Garlic cloves, minced | 1 – 2 | 1 – 2 |
| Chopped or torn romaine lettuce, lightly packed | 6 cups | 1.5 L |
| Grated daikon radish | 1 cup | 250 mL |
| Grated carrot | 1/2 cup | 125 mL |
| Coarsely chopped fresh basil | 1/2 cup | 125 mL |

Preheat barbecue to medium-high (see Note). Poke holes in steak with fork. Spread chili paste on each side of steak. Set aside.

**Sesame Lime Dressing:** Combine next 5 ingredients in small cup. Makes about 1/4 cup (60 mL) dressing.

Arrange remaining 4 ingredients on 4 salad plates. Cook steak on greased grill for 3 to 5 minutes per side until desired doneness. Transfer to cutting board. Let stand for 5 minutes. Cut steak into 1/8 inch (3 mm) wide strips. Arrange strips on each salad. Drizzle with dressing. Serves 4.

*1 serving: 304 Calories; 20.1 g Total Fat (8.1 g Mono, 3.4 g Poly, 6.1 g Sat); 47 mg Cholesterol; 12 g Carbohydrate; 1 g Fibre; 19 g Protein; 301 mg Sodium*

Pictured on page 53.

**Note:** Too cold to barbecue? Steak can be placed on a greased broiling pan and broiled on top rack in oven for 3 to 5 minutes per side until desired doneness.

# Thai Cucumber Salad

*Fresh-tasting with a touch of heat—you would expect nothing less from a Thai salad! Goes great with roasted meats.*

| | | |
|---|---|---|
| English cucumber, peeled, quartered lengthwise and cut diagonally into 1/2 inch (12 mm) pieces | 1 | 1 |
| Medium tomatoes, cut into 8 wedges each and halved | 2 | 2 |
| Green onions, cut into 1/2 inch (12 mm) pieces | 4 | 4 |
| Chopped fresh cilantro | 2 tbsp. | 30 mL |
| **PEPPY LIME DRESSING** | | |
| Lime juice | 3 tbsp. | 50 mL |
| Soy sauce | 1 tbsp. | 15 mL |
| Granulated sugar | 1 tbsp. | 15 mL |
| Cayenne pepper | 1/8 tsp. | 0.5 mL |

Put first 4 ingredients into large bowl.

**Peppy Lime Dressing:** Whisk all 4 ingredients in small bowl until combined. Makes about 1/4 cup (60 mL) dressing. Drizzle over salad. Toss. Serves 4.

*1 serving: 48 Calories; 0.4 g Total Fat (trace Mono, 0.1 g Poly, 0.1 g Sat); 0 mg Cholesterol; 11 g Carbohydrate; 2 g Fibre; 2 g Protein; 339 mg Sodium*

Pictured on page 107.

---

## Paré Pointer

*The pony had a hard time talking. He was a little hoarse.*

# Shrimp Avocado Salad

*"Pretty in pink" shrimp top a bed of crisp greens. This attractive salad is sure to please!*

| | | |
|---|---|---|
| Lime juice | 1/3 cup | 75 mL |
| Chopped fresh cilantro or parsley | 1/4 cup | 60 mL |
| Olive oil | 1 tbsp. | 15 mL |
| Jalapeño pepper, finely diced (see Tip, page 114) | 1 | 1 |
| Garlic and herb no-salt seasoning | 1 tsp. | 5 mL |
| Water | 4 cups | 1 L |
| Garlic and herb no-salt seasoning | 1 tsp. | 5 mL |
| Frozen uncooked medium shrimp (peeled and deveined), thawed | 1 lb. | 454 g |
| Chopped or torn romaine lettuce, lightly packed | 4 cups | 1 L |
| Diced fresh tomato | 1 cup | 250 mL |
| Medium avocados, cut into 8 slices each | 2 | 2 |
| Sliced green onion | 1/4 cup | 60 mL |

Combine first 5 ingredients in medium bowl.

Combine water and seasoning in medium saucepan. Bring to a boil. Add shrimp. Cook for about 2 minutes until shrimp turn pink. Drain. Rinse with cold water. Drain. Add to lime juice mixture. Stir.

Arrange next 3 ingredients, in order given, on 4 individual serving plates. Spoon shrimp mixture over top.

Sprinkle with green onion. Serves 4.

*1 serving: 301 Calories; 20.6 g Total Fat (2.8 g Mono, 1.2 g Poly, 2.1 g Sat); 172 mg Cholesterol; 12 g Carbohydrate; 5 g Fibre; 27 g Protein; 180 mg Sodium*

Pictured on page 53.

# Lean Chef's Salad

*Eat enough of this salad and you'll be a lean chef too! Consider it a full meal deal with plenty of meat, cheese and eggs.*

| | | |
|---|---|---|
| Chopped or torn romaine lettuce, lightly packed | 4 cups | 1 L |
| Green onion, sliced | 1 | 1 |
| Cherry tomatoes, halved | 8 | 8 |
| Fat-free Italian dressing | 1/3 cup | 75 mL |
| Pepper, sprinkle | | |
| Diced light medium Cheddar cheese | 1/2 cup | 125 mL |
| No-fat deli ham slices, cut into thin strips | 3 oz. | 85 g |
| Lean deli smoked turkey breast slices, cut into thin strips | 3 oz. | 85 g |
| Large hard-cooked eggs, chopped (see Note) | 2 | 2 |
| Fat-free Italian dressing (optional) | 2 tbsp. | 30 mL |

Put first 3 ingredients into large bowl. Drizzle with first amount of dressing. Sprinkle with pepper. Toss well. Arrange on two individual serving plates.

Arrange next 3 ingredients over lettuce mixture.

Sprinkle eggs over top.

Serve with second amount of dressing on the side. Serves 2.

*1 serving: 328 Calories; 14.9 g Total Fat (2.2 g Mono, 1.0 g Poly, 7.3 g Sat); 277 mg Cholesterol; 16 g Carbohydrate; 3 g Fibre; 36 g Protein; 1878 mg Sodium*

Pictured on page 53.

**Note:** Reserve 1 cooked egg yolk before chopping eggs. Use to garnish assembled salads by pressing egg yolk with a spoon through a sieve held over the salad.

# Beet And Walnut Salad

*This tempting salad beets all others! An uncomplicated salad perfectly enhanced by creamy dressing and a generous amount of walnuts.*

### CREAMY GOAT CHEESE DRESSING

| | | |
|---|---|---|
| Light mayonnaise | 2 tbsp. | 30 mL |
| Goat (chèvre) cheese, softened | 2 tbsp. | 30 mL |
| Orange juice | 2 tbsp. | 30 mL |
| Dried dillweed | 1/8 tsp. | 0.5 mL |

### SALAD

| | | |
|---|---|---|
| Mixed salad greens, lightly packed | 6 cups | 1.5 L |
| Can of sliced beets, drained and quartered (see Tip, page 47) | 14 oz. | 398 mL |
| Walnut halves, toasted (see Tip, page 14) | 1 cup | 250 mL |

**Creamy Goat Cheese Dressing:** Combine first 4 ingredients in small bowl. Makes about 1/3 cup (75 mL) dressing.

**Salad:** Combine remaining 3 ingredients in large bowl. Add dressing. Toss well. Serves 4.

*1 serving: 249 Calories; 20.1 g Total Fat (2.5 g Mono, 12.0 g Poly, 2.7 g Sat); 5 mg Cholesterol; 15 g Carbohydrate; 6 g Fibre; 7 g Protein; 291 mg Sodium*

1. Grilled Beef Salad, page 48
2. Shrimp Avocado Salad, page 50
3. Lean Chef's Salad, page 51

Props courtesy of: Cherison Enterprises Inc.
Mikasa Home Store
Pfaltzgraff Canada

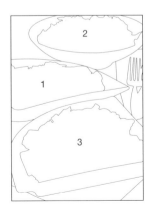

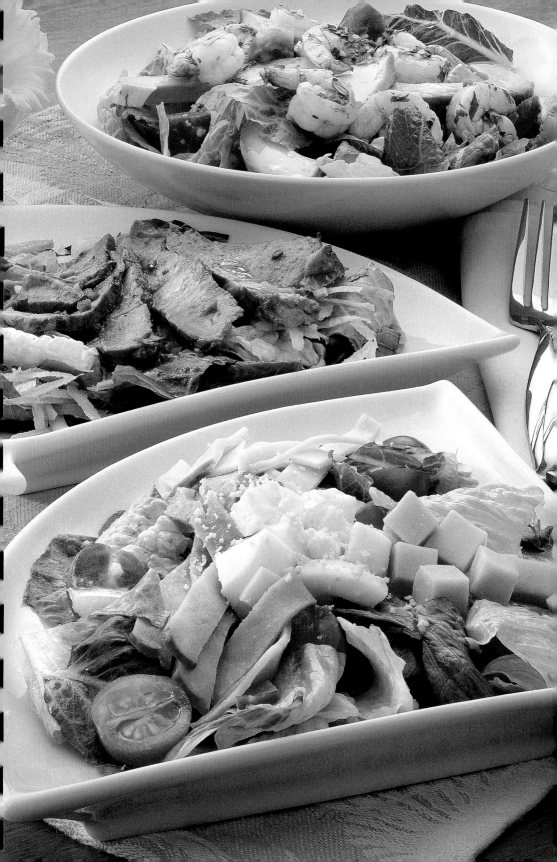

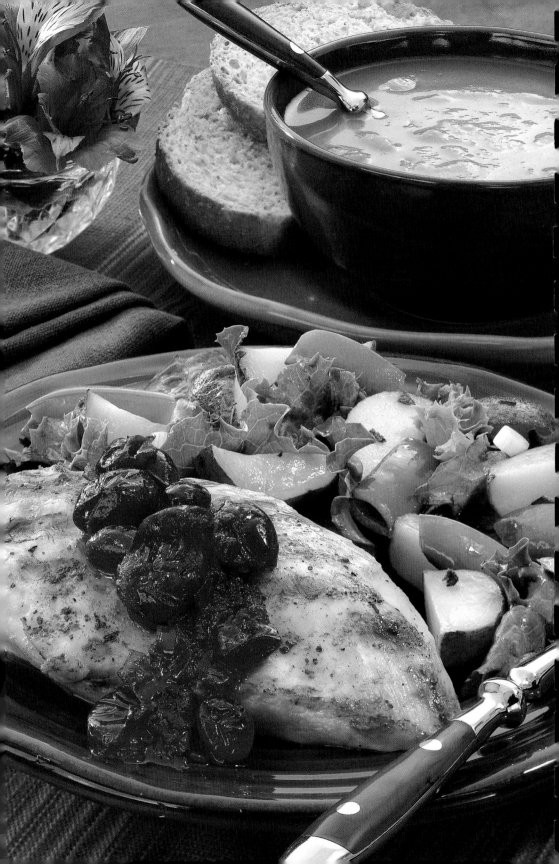

# Autumn Pumpkin Soup

*The perfect blend of pumpkin and spices! This thick pumpkin and apple soup is just what you need on a chilly fall day. Serve with slices of whole-wheat bread.*

| | | |
|---|---|---|
| Olive (or canola) oil | 2 tsp. | 10 mL |
| Chopped onion | 1 1/2 cups | 375 mL |
| Low-sodium prepared chicken (or vegetable) broth | 4 cups | 1 L |
| Can of pure pumpkin (no spices) | 14 oz. | 398 mL |
| Unsweetened applesauce | 1 cup | 250 mL |
| Bay leaf | 1 | 1 |
| Chopped fresh thyme (or 1/2 tsp., 2 mL, dried) | 2 tsp. | 10 mL |
| Lemon pepper | 1 tsp. | 5 mL |
| Salt, sprinkle | | |

Heat olive oil in large saucepan on medium. Add onion. Cook for 5 to 10 minutes, stirring occasionally, until softened and starting to brown.

Add remaining 7 ingredients. Stir. Bring to a boil. Reduce heat to medium-low. Simmer, partially covered, for 10 minutes to blend flavours. Discard bay leaf. Makes about 7 cups (1.75 L).

*1 cup (250 mL): 72 Calories; 1.9 g Total Fat (1.2 g Mono, 0.2 g Poly, 0.4 g Sat); 0 mg Cholesterol; 13 g Carbohydrate; 3 g Fibre; 2 g Protein; 42 mg Sodium*

Pictured at left.

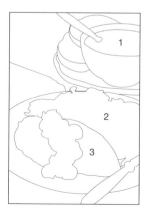

1. Autumn Pumpkin Soup, above
2. Baby Potato Sage Toss, page 47
3. Cranberry-Topped Chicken, page 82

Props courtesy of:  Cherison Enterprises Inc.
Danesco Inc.
Dansk Gifts

# Potato Pear Soup

*Nothing com-pears! Different and delicious—not your everyday potato soup. Leek and lemon enhance sweet pear to give this soup an interesting elegance.*

| | | |
|---|---|---|
| Olive oil | 2 tsp. | 10 mL |
| Chopped peeled pear | 3 cups | 750 mL |
| Sliced leek (white part only) | 1 cup | 250 mL |
| Chopped peeled potato | 3 cups | 750 mL |
| Low-sodium prepared chicken broth | 3 cups | 750 mL |
| Pepper | 1/8 tsp. | 0.5 mL |
| Lemon juice | 1 tbsp. | 15 mL |
| Grated lemon zest | 1/2 tsp. | 2 mL |

Heat olive oil in large saucepan on medium. Add pear and leek. Cook for about 5 minutes, stirring often, until leek is softened.

Add next 3 ingredients. Stir. Bring to a boil. Reduce heat to medium-low. Simmer, covered, for about 10 minutes until potato is soft. Carefully process with hand blender or in blender until smooth (see Safety Tip).

Stir in lemon juice and lemon zest. Makes about 6 cups (1.5 L).

*1 cup (250 mL): 148 Calories; 2.1 g Total Fat (1.3 g Mono, 0.3 g Poly, 0.3 g Sat); 0 mg Cholesterol; 31 g Carbohydrate; 4 g Fibre; 3 g Protein; 26 mg Sodium*

**Safety Tip:** Follow manufacturer's instructions for processing hot liquids.

# Avocado Gazpacho

*The soup is chilled but the heat's still in the spicy broth that surrounds chunks of cool avocado. Chilled vegetable cocktail ensures soup is cold and ready to serve. Try it with chopped fresh cilantro.*

| | | |
|---|---|---|
| Low-sodium vegetable cocktail juice, chilled | 2 cups | 500 mL |
| Coarsely chopped green pepper | 1/2 cup | 125 mL |
| Coarsely chopped English cucumber | 1/2 cup | 125 mL |
| Coarsely chopped green onion | 2 tbsp. | 30 mL |
| Lemon juice | 2 tbsp. | 30 mL |
| Red wine vinegar | 2 tsp. | 10 mL |
| Worcestershire sauce | 1/2 tsp. | 2 mL |

*(continued on next page)*

Soups

| Hot pepper sauce | 1/4 tsp. | 1 mL |
| Diced avocado | 1 cup | 250 mL |

Process first 8 ingredients in blender or food processor until smooth. Pour into 2 serving bowls. Makes about 3 cups (750 mL) soup.

Spoon avocado into bowls. Stir. Serves 2.

*1 serving: 189 Calories; 11.1 g Total Fat (7.4 g Mono, 1.4 g Poly, 1.6 g Sat); trace Cholesterol; 22 g Carbohydrate; 8 g Fibre; 3 g Protein; 174 mg Sodium*

---

# Quick Carrot Soup

*If carrots help your vision, then it's easy to see that this soup is an excellent choice! Orange juice and honey make this treat all the sweeter.*

| Canola (or olive) oil | 2 tsp. | 10 mL |
| Baby carrots, coarsely chopped | 1 lb. | 454 g |
| Chopped onion | 1/2 cup | 125 mL |
| Low-sodium prepared chicken broth | 3 cups | 750 mL |
| Chopped fresh dill | 1 tbsp. | 15 mL |
| (or 3/4 tsp., 4 mL, dried) | | |
| No-salt seasoning | 1 1/2 tsp. | 7 mL |
| Orange juice | 1/4 cup | 60 mL |
| Chopped fresh dill | 1 tbsp. | 15 mL |
| (or 3/4 tsp., 4 mL, dried) | | |
| Liquid honey | 1 tbsp. | 15 mL |

Heat canola oil in large saucepan on medium. Add carrot and onion. Cook for about 10 minutes, stirring occasionally, until onion is softened.

Add next 3 ingredients. Bring to a boil. Reduce heat to medium-low. Simmer, uncovered, for about 5 minutes until carrot is tender. Carefully process with hand blender or in blender until smooth (see Safety Tip).

Add remaining 3 ingredients. Cook on medium for about 1 minute, stirring occasionally, until heated through. Makes about 4 1/2 cups (1.1 L).

*1 cup (250 mL): 107 Calories; 2.5 g Total Fat (1.4 g Mono, 0.7 g Poly, 0.3 g Sat); 0 mg Cholesterol; 19 g Carbohydrate; 3 g Fibre; 3 g Protein; 78 mg Sodium*

**Safety Tip:** Follow manufacturer's instructions for processing hot liquids.

# Sweet Pea Soup

*Not to worry, we don't expect you to sup on your garden flora—it's the peas that impart a sweet flavour. Great on its own, but sensational with the creamy Minted Yogurt topping.*

| | | |
|---|---|---|
| Olive (or canola) oil | 2 tsp. | 10 mL |
| Finely chopped green onion | 1/2 cup | 125 mL |
| Garlic clove, minced | 1 | 1 |
| (or 1/4 tsp., 1 mL, powder) | | |
| Frozen peas | 2 cups | 500 mL |
| Chopped or torn green leaf lettuce, | 1 1/2 cups | 375 mL |
| lightly packed | | |
| Low-sodium prepared chicken | 3 cups | 750 mL |
| (or vegetable) broth | | |
| Pepper | 1/4 tsp. | 1 mL |
| Frozen peas | 1/2 cup | 125 mL |
| MINTED YOGURT | | |
| Plain yogurt | 1/3 cup | 75 mL |
| Chopped fresh mint | 2 tbsp. | 30 mL |

Heat olive oil in medium saucepan on medium. Add green onion and garlic. Cook for about 5 minutes, stirring occasionally, until green onion is softened.

Add first amount of peas and lettuce. Heat and stir for 1 minute. Add broth and pepper. Bring to a boil. Reduce heat to medium-low. Simmer for 3 to 5 minutes, stirring occasionally, until peas are tender. Carefully process with hand blender or in blender until smooth (see Safety Tip).

Add second amount of peas. Heat and stir on medium for about 2 minutes until peas are tender. Makes about 4 1/2 cups (1.1 L) soup.

**Minted Yogurt:** Combine yogurt and mint in small bowl. Makes about 6 tbsp. (100 mL) yogurt. Spoon onto individual servings. Serves 4.

*1 serving: 126 Calories; 3.8 g Total Fat (2.1 g Mono, 0.5 g Poly, 0.9 g Sat); 3 mg Cholesterol; 16 g Carbohydrate; 5 g Fibre; 8 g Protein; 144 mg Sodium*

Pictured on page 143.

**Safety Tip:** Follow manufacturer's instructions for processing hot liquids.

# Zucchini Dill Soup

*Kitchen overflowing with a fall harvest of zucchini? Put that bounty to good use in this easy-to-make, creamy soup with a subtle flavouring of dill. Garnish with fresh dill sprigs.*

| | | |
|---|---|---|
| Canola oil | 2 tsp. | 10 mL |
| Sliced zucchini | 3 cups | 750 mL |
| Chopped onion | 3/4 cup | 175 mL |
| Sliced celery | 3/4 cup | 175 mL |
| All-purpose flour | 2 tbsp. | 30 mL |
| Dried dillweed | 1/2 tsp. | 2 mL |
| Pepper | 1/8 tsp. | 0.5 mL |
| Low-sodium prepared chicken broth | 2 cups | 500 mL |
| Milk | 1 1/2 cups | 375 mL |

Heat canola oil in large saucepan on medium-high. Add next 3 ingredients. Cook for about 8 minutes, stirring often, until onion and celery are softened and starting to brown.

Sprinkle next 3 ingredients over zucchini mixture. Heat and stir for 1 minute.

Add 1 cup (250 mL) broth. Heat and stir until boiling and thickened. Add remaining broth and milk. Bring to a boil. Reduce heat to medium-low. Simmer for 5 minutes to blend flavours. Carefully process with hand blender or in blender until smooth (see Safety Tip). Makes about 5 cups (1.25 L).

*1 cup (250 mL): 93 Calories; 3.2 g Total Fat (1.5 g Mono, 0.7 g Poly, 0.8 g Sat); 3 mg Cholesterol; 12 g Carbohydrate; 1 g Fibre; 5 g Protein; 79 mg Sodium*

**Safety Tip:** Follow manufacturer's instructions for processing hot liquids.

## Paré Pointer

*The wheels on a car are always tired.*

# Chicken Bean Soup

*There's certainly nothing wrong with being full of beans—when you're talking about a soup! This veggie-packed chicken soup has just a hint of cayenne heat. Perfect when you're feeling under the weather.*

| | | |
|---|---|---|
| Olive oil | 2 tsp. | 10 mL |
| Chopped onion | 1 cup | 250 mL |
| Chopped carrot | 2/3 cup | 150 mL |
| Chopped celery | 1/2 cup | 125 mL |
| Low-sodium prepared chicken broth | 8 cups | 2 L |
| Diced peeled potato | 1 1/2 cups | 375 mL |
| Paprika | 1 1/2 tsp. | 7 mL |
| Cayenne pepper, sprinkle | | |
| Can of navy beans, rinsed and drained | 14 oz. | 398 mL |
| Chopped cooked chicken | 1 cup | 250 mL |

Heat olive oil in large saucepan or Dutch oven on medium-high. Add next 3 ingredients. Cook for about 5 minutes, stirring often, until onion starts to brown.

Add next 4 ingredients. Stir. Bring to a boil. Reduce heat to medium. Boil gently, partially covered, for about 10 minutes until potato is softened.

Add beans and chicken. Stir. Cook for about 2 minutes until heated through. Makes about 10 cups (2.5 L).

*1 cup (250 mL): 135 Calories; 2.7 g Total Fat (1.3 g Mono, 0.6 g Poly, 0.6 g Sat); 11 mg Cholesterol; 19 g Carbohydrate; 4 g Fibre; 10 g Protein; 145 mg Sodium*

# Chicken Yam Chowder

*Your family will be yammering for more! Yams replace traditional potatoes in this chicken corn chowder with a southwestern twist.*

| | | |
|---|---|---|
| Large unpeeled yam (or sweet potato) (about 1 1/2 lbs., 680 g), see Note | 1 | 1 |
| Canola oil | 2 tsp. | 10 mL |
| Diced onion | 1 cup | 250 mL |
| Diced green pepper | 1 cup | 250 mL |
| Low-sodium prepared chicken broth | 4 cups | 1 L |
| Chopped cooked chicken | 2 cups | 500 mL |
| Frozen kernel corn | 1 cup | 250 mL |
| Chunky salsa | 1/2 cup | 125 mL |
| Chopped fresh oregano (or 1/4 tsp., 1 mL, dried) | 1 tsp. | 5 mL |
| No-salt seasoning | 1 tsp. | 5 mL |
| Can of evaporated milk | 5 1/2 oz. | 160 mL |

Cut yam in half lengthwise. Microwave, covered, on high (100%), for about 8 minutes until tender. Remove pulp to medium bowl. Mash with fork. Discard peel.

Meanwhile, heat canola oil in large saucepan on medium. Add onion and green pepper. Cook for 5 to 10 minutes, stirring occasionally, until softened.

Add yam and next 6 ingredients. Bring to a boil. Reduce heat to medium. Boil gently, partially covered, for 5 minutes to blend flavours.

Add evaporated milk. Heat and stir until hot, but not boiling. Makes about 9 cups (2.25 L).

*1 cup (250 mL): 201 Calories; 5.4 g Total Fat (2.1 g Mono, 1.1 g Poly, 1.8 g Sat); 32 mg Cholesterol; 26 g Carbohydrate; 4 g Fibre; 13 g Protein; 184 mg Sodium*

**Note:** You can make this soup even more quickly by using 3 cups (750 mL) of mashed canned sweet potato. The microwave cooking time for the yam is then eliminated.

# Turkey Minestrone

*A hearty, meal-style soup. Not too spicy, but very flavourful. Freeze in individual portions and take for lunch.*

| | | |
|---|---|---|
| Olive oil | 2 tsp. | 10 mL |
| Extra-lean ground turkey | 3/4 lb. | 340 g |
| Finely chopped onion | 3/4 cup | 175 mL |
| Finely chopped celery | 3/4 cup | 175 mL |
| Garlic cloves, minced | 2 | 2 |
| (or 1/2 tsp., 2 mL, powder) | | |
| Italian seasoning | 1 tsp. | 5 mL |
| Low-sodium prepared chicken broth | 6 cups | 1.5 L |
| Can of white kidney beans, rinsed and drained | 19 oz. | 540 mL |
| Can of diced tomatoes (with juice) | 14 oz. | 398 mL |
| Whole-wheat elbow macaroni | 1/2 cup | 125 mL |
| Frozen cut green beans | 1 cup | 250 mL |
| Chopped fresh oregano | 1 tbsp. | 15 mL |
| (or 3/4 tsp., 4 mL, dried) | | |
| Chopped fresh sage | 1 1/2 tsp. | 7 mL |
| (or 1/4 tsp., 1 mL, dried) | | |

Heat olive oil in large saucepan or Dutch oven on medium-high. Add next 5 ingredients. Scramble-fry for 5 to 10 minutes until turkey is no longer pink and vegetables are tender.

Add next 4 ingredients. Bring to a boil. Reduce heat to medium. Boil gently, partially covered, for 8 to 10 minutes, stirring occasionally, until macaroni is tender but firm.

Add remaining 3 ingredients. Cook for about 2 minutes until beans are tender-crisp. Makes about 10 cups (2.5 L).

*1 cup (250 mL): 143 Calories; 4.0 g Total Fat (0.9 g Mono, 0.2 g Poly, 0.9 g Sat); 19 mg Cholesterol; 16 g Carbohydrate; 3 g Fibre; 12 g Protein; 199 mg Sodium*

 *fyi* Tomatoes are a great source of lycopene, a powerful antioxidant. And believe it or not, lycopene is actually more potent when the tomatoes are cooked.

# Curried Vegetable Soup

*This is one curry that's ready in a hurry—and will disappear in a hurry, too!*
*This thick puréed soup with a medium level of curry heat is nicely balanced*
*with sweet vegetables.*

| | | |
|---|---|---|
| Canola oil | 2 tsp. | 10 mL |
| Chopped onion | 1 cup | 250 mL |
| Chopped carrot | 1 cup | 250 mL |
| Chopped celery | 1 cup | 250 mL |
| Granulated sugar | 4 tsp. | 20 mL |
| Curry powder | 2 tsp. | 10 mL |
| Garlic cloves, minced | 2 | 2 |
| (or 1/2 tsp., 2 mL, powder) | | |
| Prepared vegetable (or chicken) broth | 4 cups | 1 L |
| Grated zucchini | 2 cups | 500 mL |
| Grated peeled potato | 1 cup | 250 mL |
| Salt | 1/4 tsp. | 1 mL |
| Pepper | 1/4 tsp. | 1 mL |
| Plain yogurt | 1/2 cup | 125 mL |

**Sliced green onion, for garnish**

Heat canola oil in large saucepan on medium-high. Add next 3 ingredients. Cook for about 3 minutes, stirring often, until vegetables start to soften.

Add next 3 ingredients. Heat and stir for about 1 minute until fragrant.

Add next 5 ingredients. Stir. Bring to a boil. Reduce heat to medium-low. Simmer, covered, for about 10 minutes until vegetables are soft. Carefully process with hand blender or in blender until smooth (see Safety Tip).

Add yogurt. Stir.

Garnish with green onion. Makes about 7 1/2 cups (1.9 L).

*1 cup (250 mL): 75 Calories; 2.0 g Total Fat (0.9 g Mono, 0.5 g Poly, 0.5 g Sat); 2 mg Cholesterol; 13 g Carbohydrate; 2 g Fibre; 2 g Protein; 602 mg Sodium*

**Safety Tip:** Follow manufacturer's instructions for processing hot liquids.

# Pepper Power Soup

*This tasty treat will give you all the "souper powers" you need to get through your day! Loaded with flavour and hearty vegetables.*

| | | |
|---|---|---|
| Olive oil | 2 tsp. | 10 mL |
| Chopped red pepper | 2 cups | 500 mL |
| Chopped onion | 1 cup | 250 mL |
| Finely diced jalapeño pepper (see Tip, page 114) | 1 tbsp. | 15 mL |
| Garlic cloves, minced | 2 | 2 |
| Low-sodium prepared chicken broth | 6 cups | 1.5 L |
| Frozen kernel corn | 2 cups | 500 mL |
| Chopped kale leaves, lightly packed (see Tip, page 110) | 2 cups | 500 mL |
| Can of diced tomatoes (with juice) | 14 oz. | 398 mL |
| Lime juice | 2 tbsp. | 30 mL |
| Chopped fresh cilantro or parsley | 3 tbsp. | 50 mL |

Heat olive oil in large saucepan or Dutch oven on medium. Add next 4 ingredients. Cook for about 5 minutes, stirring occasionally, until red pepper is softened.

Add next 5 ingredients. Stir. Bring to a boil. Reduce heat to medium-low. Simmer, partially covered, for about 15 minutes until kale is tender.

Add cilantro. Stir. Makes about 10 1/2 cups (2.6 L).

*1 cup (250 mL): 75 Calories; 1.7 g Total Fat (0.9 g Mono, 0.4 g Poly, 0.3 g Sat); 0 mg Cholesterol; 14 g Carbohydrate; 2 g Fibre; 4 g Protein; 132 mg Sodium*

**Variation:** Use same amount of chopped fresh spinach leaves instead of chopped kale. Reduce simmering time to 5 minutes.

 Let's raise our glasses and make a toast to red wine. Drinking it in moderation actually improves cardiovascular health (how often can you say that about something many of us consider an indulgence?). If you choose not to imbibe alcohol, opt for a non-alcoholic red wine—it offers similar benefits.

# Curry Chicken Vegetable Soup

*Perfect for a cold wintry day! A quick and warming soup filled with chicken and vegetables. Tastes just like mulligatawny without the rice. Curry lovers can add a smidgeon more to increase the heat level.*

| | | |
|---|---|---|
| Canola oil | 1 1/2 tsp. | 7 mL |
| Finely chopped celery | 3/4 cup | 175 mL |
| Finely chopped onion | 3/4 cup | 175 mL |
| Medium cooking apple (such as McIntosh), peeled and grated | 1 | 1 |
| All-purpose flour | 2 tbsp. | 30 mL |
| Curry powder | 1 tsp. | 5 mL |
| Salt | 1/4 tsp. | 1 mL |
| Cayenne pepper | 1/8 tsp. | 0.5 mL |
| Low-sodium prepared chicken broth | 5 cups | 1.25 L |
| Chopped cooked chicken | 1 1/2 cups | 375 mL |
| Frozen mixed vegetables | 1 1/2 cups | 375 mL |
| Lemon juice | 1 tbsp. | 15 mL |

Heat canola oil in large saucepan on medium. Add celery and onion. Cook for about 3 minutes, stirring occasionally, until starting to soften.

Add next 5 ingredients. Heat and stir for 1 minute.

Add 1 cup (250 mL) broth. Heat and stir until boiling and thickened. Add remaining broth, chicken and vegetables. Bring to a boil. Reduce heat to medium-low. Simmer, uncovered, for 8 minutes to blend flavours.

Add lemon juice. Stir. Makes about 7 1/2 cups (1.9 L).

*1 cup (250 mL): 94 Calories; 2.7 g Total Fat (1.2 g Mono, 0.7 g Poly, 0.6 g Sat); 14 mg Cholesterol; 10 g Carbohydrate; 2 g Fibre; 7 g Protein; 149 mg Sodium*

# Speedy Beef Ragout

*With just a little thyme, you'll have an attractive and appetizing stew! Serve with crusty rolls or slices of whole-wheat French bread.*

| | | |
|---|---|---|
| All-purpose flour | 2 tbsp. | 30 mL |
| Seasoned salt | 1/2 tsp. | 2 mL |
| Pepper | 1 tsp. | 5 mL |
| Beef stir-fry strips | 1 lb. | 454 g |
| Canola oil | 1 tbsp. | 15 mL |
| Canola oil | 1 tsp. | 5 mL |
| Sliced fresh white mushrooms | 2 cups | 500 mL |
| Chopped onion | 1 cup | 250 mL |
| Thinly sliced carrot | 3/4 cup | 175 mL |
| Garlic cloves, minced | 2 | 2 |
| (or 1/2 tsp., 2 mL, powder) | | |
| Dried thyme | 1 tsp. | 5 mL |
| All-purpose flour | 1 tsp. | 5 mL |
| Prepared beef broth | 1 1/2 cups | 375 mL |
| Red wine vinegar | 1 tbsp. | 15 mL |
| Chopped fresh parsley | 2 tbsp. | 30 mL |

Measure first 3 ingredients into large resealable freezer bag. Add beef. Seal bag. Toss until coated.

Heat first amount of canola oil in large frying pan on medium-high. Add beef. Cook for 3 to 4 minutes, stirring often, until browned. Transfer to medium bowl. Cover to keep warm.

Heat second amount of canola oil in same frying pan. Add next 5 ingredients. Cook for about 2 minutes, stirring occasionally, until vegetables start to soften.

Add second amount of flour. Heat and stir for 1 minute.

Add broth and vinegar. Stir. Bring to a boil. Reduce heat to medium. Boil gently, covered, for about 10 minutes until vegetables are tender. Add beef. Heat and stir for 1 to 2 minutes until heated through. Transfer to large serving dish.

Sprinkle with parsley. Makes about 4 cups (1 L).

*1 cup (250 mL): 356 Calories; 22.1 g Total Fat (10.1 g Mono, 2.1 g Poly, 7.4 g Sat); 62 mg Cholesterol; 12 g Carbohydrate; 2 g Fibre; 27 g Protein; 515 mg Sodium*

# Ginger Beef

*The usual deep-fried breading is eliminated in this unique version of the takeout staple—but fear not, it's just as tasty.*

| | | |
|---|---|---|
| Water | 2 1/4 cups | 550 mL |
| Converted white rice | 1 cup | 250 mL |
| Salt (optional) | 1/4 tsp. | 1 mL |
| Prepared beef broth | 1/4 cup | 60 mL |
| Medium sherry | 2 tbsp. | 30 mL |
| Soy sauce | 2 tbsp. | 30 mL |
| Cornstarch | 1 tbsp. | 15 mL |
| Finely grated ginger root | 1 tbsp. | 15 mL |
| Brown sugar, packed | 1 tbsp. | 15 mL |
| Garlic clove, minced | 1 | 1 |
| Dried crushed chilies | 1/4 tsp. | 1 mL |
| Canola oil | 2 tsp. | 10 mL |
| Beef stir-fry strips | 1 lb. | 454 g |
| Sliced onion | 1/2 cup | 125 mL |
| Bag of frozen California mixed vegetables, thawed (see Tip, below) | 1 lb. | 454 g |

Sesame seeds, for garnish

Measure first 3 ingredients into medium saucepan. Bring to a boil. Reduce heat to medium-low. Simmer, covered, for about 20 minutes, without stirring, until water is absorbed and rice is tender.

Meanwhile, combine next 8 ingredients in small bowl. Set aside.

Heat wok or large frying pan on medium-high until very hot. Add canola oil. Add beef and onion. Stir-fry for 4 minutes.

Add vegetables and broth mixture. Stir-fry for about 3 minutes until vegetables are tender-crisp and sauce is boiling and thickened. Fluff rice with fork. Spoon into 4 individual serving bowls. Spoon beef mixture over rice.

Garnish with sesame seeds. Serves 4.

*1 serving: 515 Calories; 19.8 g Total Fat (8.8 g Mono, 1.5 g Poly, 7.2 g Sat); 62 mg Cholesterol; 52 g Carbohydrate; 4 g Fibre; 30 g Protein; 597 mg Sodium*

 *tip* To quickly thaw frozen vegetables, rinse under cool water or defrost in the microwave.

# Beef Bourguignon Patties

*You're never bourgeois when you're eating bourguignon (pronounced boor-gee-NYON)! You'll feel simply aristocratic when you nosh on beef patties in a delicious mushroom and wine sauce. Serve with egg noodles or mashed potatoes.*

| | | |
|---|---|---|
| Egg white (large) | 1 | 1 |
| Fine dry bread crumbs | 3/4 cup | 175 mL |
| Natural wheat bran | 1/4 cup | 60 mL |
| Dijon mustard | 2 tbsp. | 30 mL |
| Pepper | 1/4 tsp. | 1 mL |
| Extra-lean (or lean) ground beef | 1 lb. | 454 g |
| Canola oil | 2 tsp. | 10 mL |
| Sliced fresh white mushrooms | 1 cup | 250 mL |
| Finely chopped onion | 1/4 cup | 60 mL |
| Dry (or alcohol-free) red wine | 1/2 cup | 125 mL |
| Low-sodium prepared beef broth | 1 cup | 250 mL |
| Tomato paste (see Tip, page 83) | 1 tbsp. | 15 mL |
| Sprig of fresh rosemary | 1/2 | 1/2 |
| Sprig of fresh thyme | 1 | 1 |
| Low-sodium prepared beef broth | 2 tbsp. | 30 mL |
| All-purpose flour | 2 tsp. | 10 mL |

Preheat broiler. Combine first 5 ingredients in large bowl. Add beef. Mix well. Divide into 4 equal portions. Shape into 1/2 inch (12 mm) thick patties. Place on greased broiling pan. Broil on centre rack in oven for about 5 minutes per side until fully cooked, and internal temperature of beef reaches 160°F (71°C).

Meanwhile, heat canola oil in large frying pan on medium-high. Add mushrooms and onion. Cook for about 4 minutes, stirring occasionally, until starting to turn golden.

Add wine. Stir. Reduce heat to medium.

Stir in next 4 ingredients. Boil gently, uncovered, for 5 minutes to blend flavours.

Stir second amount of beef broth and flour in small cup until smooth. Add to mushroom mixture. Heat and stir for about 2 minutes until sauce is boiling and thickened. Add patties. Cook for 2 to 3 minutes until heated through. Discard sprigs of rosemary and thyme. Serves 4.

*1 serving: 288 Calories; 8.1 g Total Fat (3.9 g Mono, 1.5 g Poly, 2.0 g Sat); 60 mg Cholesterol; 21 g Carbohydrate; 3 g Fibre; 28 g Protein; 363 mg Sodium*

# Mushroom Steak Sandwiches

*You'll be strong to the finish when you sneak in your spinach (into this yummy deli-style sandwich). A uniquely upscale take on an old favourite.*

| | | |
|---|---|---|
| Sliced fresh white mushrooms | 2 cups | 500 mL |
| Garlic clove, minced | 1 | 1 |
| (or 1/4 tsp., 1 mL, powder) | | |
| Montreal steak spice | 1/4 tsp. | 1 mL |
| Montreal steak spice | 1/2 tsp. | 2 mL |
| Beef strip loin steak | 1 lb. | 454 g |
| Light mayonnaise | 2 tbsp. | 30 mL |
| Sesame (or canola) oil | 1 tbsp. | 15 mL |
| Finely grated ginger root | 1/2 tsp. | 2 mL |
| (or 1/8 tsp., 0.5 mL, ground ginger) | | |
| Chopped fresh spinach leaves, lightly packed | 2 cups | 500 mL |
| Whole-wheat kaiser rolls, split | 4 | 4 |

Preheat gas barbecue to medium-high. Place mushrooms and garlic on 18 inch (45 cm) long sheet of heavy-duty (or double layer of regular) foil. Sprinkle with first amount of steak spice. Fold edges of foil together over mushrooms to enclose. Fold ends to seal completely. Place on grill.

Sprinkle second amount of steak spice on steak. Cook on greased grill for 4 to 5 minutes per side until desired doneness. Transfer to cutting board. Let stand for 5 minutes. Cut steak crosswise into 1/8 inch (3 mm) slices. Remove mushroom packet from grill.

Meanwhile, combine next 3 ingredients in small bowl. Add spinach. Toss.

Arrange spinach mixture on bottom halves of rolls. Arrange steak slices over spinach. Spoon mushrooms over steak. Cover with top halves of rolls. Makes 4 sandwiches.

*1 sandwich:* 494 Calories; 29.0 g Total Fat (10.8 g Mono, 3.4 g Poly, 9.6 g Sat); 79 mg Cholesterol; 32 g Carbohydrate; 5 g Fibre; 28 g Protein; 534 mg Sodium

Pictured on page 71 and on back cover.

# Moroccan Steaks

*Grilled steaks with an exotic flair. Cinnamon, cumin and olives make this dish de-lish!*

| | | |
|---|---|---|
| Orange juice | 3 tbsp. | 50 mL |
| Tomato paste (see Tip, page 83) | 1 tbsp. | 15 mL |
| Olive oil | 1 tbsp. | 15 mL |
| Garlic powder | 1/2 tsp. | 2 mL |
| Ground cinnamon | 1/2 tsp. | 2 mL |
| Ground cumin | 1/2 tsp. | 2 mL |
| Beef strip loin steaks, halved crosswise (about 8 oz., 225 g, each) | 2 | 2 |
| Large red peppers, cut into 1/2 inch (12 mm) rings | 2 | 2 |
| Salt, sprinkle | | |
| Pepper, sprinkle | | |
| Can of sliced black olives, drained | 4 1/2 oz. | 125 mL |

Preheat gas barbecue to medium-high (see Note). Combine first 6 ingredients in small cup.

Brush orange juice mixture on 1 side of steaks and both sides of red pepper. Sprinkle steaks with salt and pepper. Cook steaks and red pepper on greased grill for 4 to 6 minutes per side, brushing once with remaining orange juice mixture, until desired doneness. Transfer steaks to serving plate.

Chop red pepper. Add to olives in small bowl. Stir. Spoon over steaks. Serves 4.

*1 serving: 352 Calories; 24.1 g Total Fat (12.3 g Mono, 1.4 g Poly, 7.8 g Sat); 62 mg Cholesterol; 10 g Carbohydrate; 3 g Fibre; 25 g Protein; 344 mg Sodium*

**Note:** Too cold to barbecue? Steaks and red pepper can be placed on a greased broiling pan and broiled on top rack in oven for 4 to 6 minutes per side until steaks and red pepper reach desired doneness.

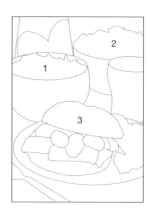

1. Apple Carrot Slaw, page 37
2. Creamy Pasta Salad, page 44
3. Mushroom Steak Sandwiches, page 69

Props courtesy of: Danesco Inc.
Anchor Hocking Canada

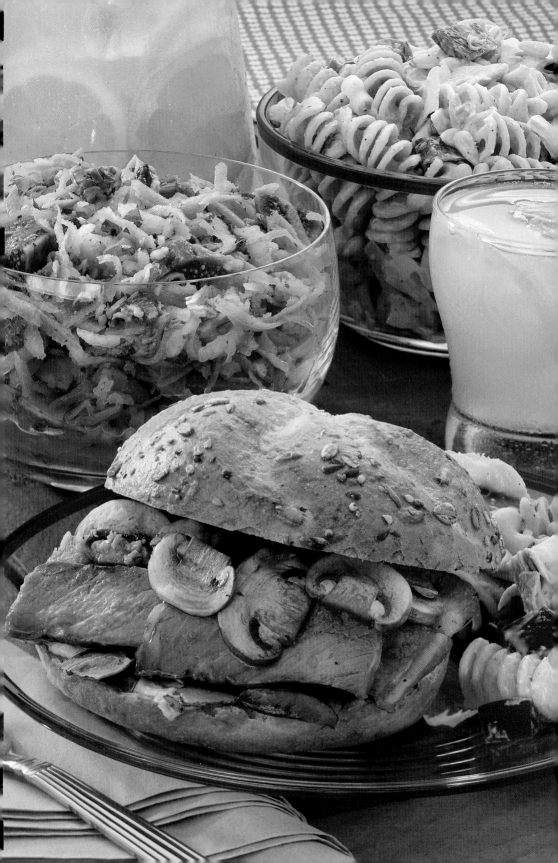

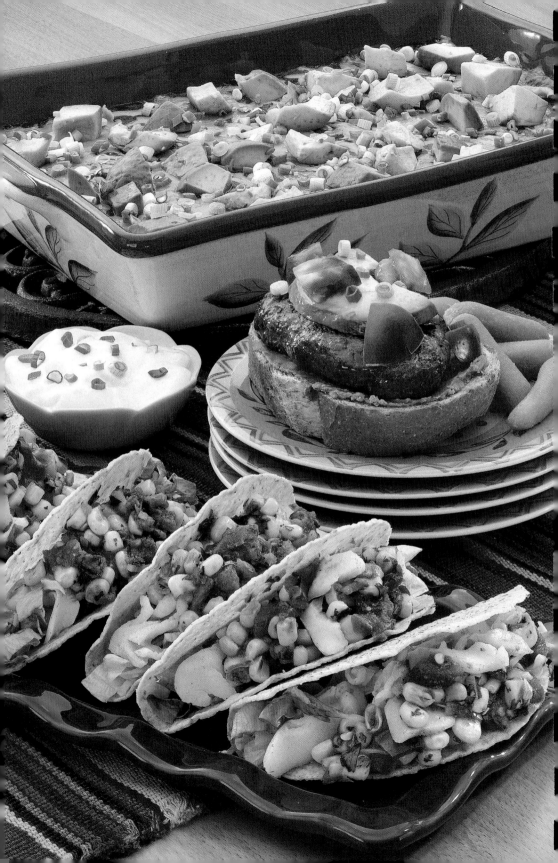

# Thai Beef Curry

*Thai-up dinner in no time with this impressive curry. Long on taste and short on cooking time.*

| | | |
|---|---|---|
| Canola oil | 2 tsp. | 10 mL |
| Thinly sliced beef top sirloin steak | 1 lb. | 454 g |
| Green onions, cut diagonally into 1 inch (2.5 cm) slices | 3 | 3 |
| Finely grated ginger root | 1 tbsp. | 15 mL |
| Garlic cloves, minced (or 1/2 tsp., 2 mL, powder) | 2 | 2 |
| Cans of cut sweet potatoes (19 oz., 540 mL, each), drained | 2 | 2 |
| Can of diced tomatoes, drained | 14 oz. | 398 mL |
| Can of light coconut milk | 14 oz. | 398 mL |
| Brown sugar, packed | 2 tbsp. | 30 mL |
| Grated lime zest (see Tip, page 140) | 1 tbsp. | 15 mL |
| Red curry paste | 1 tsp. | 5 mL |
| Lime juice | 1 tbsp. | 15 mL |

Heat canola oil in large frying pan on medium-high. Add next 4 ingredients. Stir-fry for 3 to 5 minutes until beef is starting to brown.

Add next 6 ingredients. Stir. Bring to a boil. Reduce heat to medium. Simmer, uncovered, for 10 minutes to blend flavours.

Add lime juice. Stir. Serves 4.

*1 serving: 643 Calories; 27.1 g Total Fat (9.0 g Mono, 1.8 g Poly, 12.7 g Sat); 62 mg Cholesterol; 71 g Carbohydrate; 8 g Fibre; 28 g Protein; 397 mg Sodium*

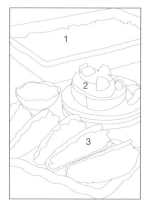

**THAI CHICKEN CURRY:** Use chicken instead of beef. Use about 4 cups (1 L) chopped fresh (or frozen) mango instead of sweet potato.

1. Enchilada Casserole, page 106
2. Open-Faced Burgers, page 74
3. Corn And Cod Tacos, page 94

Props courtesy of: Cherison Enterprises Inc.
Emile Henry

Beef

# Open-Faced Burgers

*Top your burgers with all the flavours of a layered bean dip. Hearty and filling, with a colourful presentation.*

| | | |
|---|---|---|
| Fine dry bread crumbs | 2 tbsp. | 30 mL |
| Chili powder | 1 tbsp. | 15 mL |
| Seasoned salt | 1/2 tsp. | 2 mL |
| Ground cumin | 1/2 tsp. | 2 mL |
| Extra-lean ground beef | 1 lb. | 454 g |
| Whole-wheat French bread slices, about 1 inch (2.5 cm) thick | 4 | 4 |
| Refried beans | 1/2 cup | 125 mL |
| Thin avocado slices (about 1/2 avocado) | 8 | 8 |
| Small tomato, chopped | 1 | 1 |
| Green onion, sliced | 1 | 1 |

Preheat gas barbecue to medium-high (see Note). Meanwhile, combine first 4 ingredients in large bowl. Add beef. Mix well. Shape into 4 oval patties to fit bread slices.

Toast bread slices on ungreased grill for about 1 minute per side until golden. Remove to plate. Cook patties on greased grill for about 5 minutes per side until fully cooked, and internal temperature of beef reaches 160°F (71°C).

Meanwhile, spread refried beans on toast. Place patties on top.

Top with avocado, tomato and green onion. Makes 4 burgers.

*1 burger: 312 Calories; 10.7 g Total Fat (5.4 g Mono, 1.6 g Poly, 2.6 g Sat); 63 mg Cholesterol; 28 g Carbohydrate; 7 g Fibre; 29 g Protein; 539 mg Sodium*

Pictured on page 72.

**Note:** Too cold to barbecue? Patties can be placed on a greased broiling pan and broiled on top rack in oven for about 5 minutes per side until fully cooked, and internal temperature of beef reaches 160°F (71°C). Bread slices can be placed on a baking sheet and broiled for about 1 minute per side until golden.

# Simple Beef Broccoli

*Don't let the name fool you—this dish's perfection is in its simplicity.*
*Use precut beef stir-fry strips to fix this dish even faster. Serve with steamed*
*rice for a complete meal.*

| | | |
|---|---|---|
| Low-sodium prepared beef broth | 3/4 cup | 175 mL |
| Cornstarch | 2 tbsp. | 30 mL |
| Low-sodium soy sauce | 2 tbsp. | 30 mL |
| Sesame oil (optional) | 1 tsp. | 5 mL |
| Canola oil | 1 tbsp. | 15 mL |
| Beef top sirloin steak, thinly sliced | 1 lb. | 454 g |
| Dry sherry | 2 tbsp. | 30 mL |
| Garlic cloves, minced | 2 | 2 |
| (or 1/2 tsp., 2 mL, powder) | | |
| Finely grated ginger root | 2 tsp. | 10 mL |
| (or 1/2 tsp., 2 mL, ground ginger) | | |
| Broccoli florets | 4 cups | 1 L |
| Sliced carrot, cut diagonally into | 1 1/4 cups | 300 mL |
| 1/8 inch (3 mm) slices | | |
| Sliced green onion, cut diagonally into | 1/2 cup | 125 mL |
| 1/2 inch (12 mm) slices | | |

Combine first 4 ingredients in small bowl. Set aside.

Heat wok or large frying pan on medium-high until very hot. Add canola oil. Add beef. Stir-fry for 2 minutes.

Add next 3 ingredients. Stir-fry for 2 minutes.

Add broccoli and carrot. Stir-fry for about 3 minutes until vegetables are tender-crisp.

Add green onion. Stir broth mixture. Add to beef mixture. Heat and stir for about 2 minutes until boiling and thickened. Serves 4.

*1 serving: 364 Calories; 22.1 g Total Fat (9.8 g Mono, 2.3 g Poly, 7.4 g Sat); 62 mg Cholesterol; 13 g Carbohydrate; 4 g Fibre; 27 g Protein; 357 mg Sodium*

Don't just eat food, eat super food! Because of its many nutritional benefits, broccoli is considered a super food. It's high in antioxidants, fibre and vitamins A and C. Other super foods are: salmon, chili peppers, spinach, mangoes, beans and oats, to name just a few.

# Chipotle Beef Skillet

*Consider it chili extraordinaire! Spicy chipotles and dark raisins give this unique taste treat a smoky, yet sweet flavour.*

| | | |
|---|---|---|
| Canola oil | 2 tsp. | 10 mL |
| Extra-lean ground beef | 1 lb. | 454 g |
| Chopped onion | 1/2 cup | 125 mL |
| All-purpose flour | 2 tbsp. | 30 mL |
| Garlic powder | 1/4 tsp. | 1 mL |
| Ground cumin | 1/4 tsp. | 1 mL |
| Pepper, sprinkle | | |
| Low-sodium prepared beef broth | 2 cups | 500 mL |
| Can of red kidney beans, rinsed and drained | 14 oz. | 398 mL |
| Dark raisins | 1/2 cup | 125 mL |
| Tomato paste (see Tip, page 83) | 1 tbsp. | 15 mL |
| Chopped chipotle peppers in adobo sauce (see Tip, below) | 1 1/2 tsp. | 7 mL |

Heat canola oil in large frying pan on medium-high. Add beef and onion. Scramble-fry for about 8 minutes until beef is no longer pink and onion is softened.

Add next 4 ingredients. Heat and stir for 1 minute.

Add 1 cup (250 mL) broth. Heat and stir until boiling and thickened. Reduce heat to medium. Add remaining broth and next 4 ingredients. Stir. Cook, uncovered, for 5 to 10 minutes, stirring occasionally. Serves 4.

*1 serving: 359 Calories; 7.8 g Total Fat (3.5 g Mono, 1.3 g Poly, 1.8 g Sat); 60 mg Cholesterol; 42 g Carbohydrate; 10 g Fibre; 32 g Protein; 88 mg Sodium*

 Chipotle chili peppers are smoked jalapeno peppers. Be sure to wash your hands after handling. To store any leftover chipotle chili peppers, divide into recipe-friendly portions and freeze, with sauce, in airtight containers for up to one year.

# Quick Beef Wraps

*That's a wrap! All your bases are covered with this mix of fresh veggies, cheese, meat, beans and fresh dill yogurt. Good food for when you're on the go!*

| | | |
|---|---|---|
| Canola oil | 2 tsp. | 10 mL |
| Extra-lean ground beef | 1 lb. | 454 g |
| Finely chopped onion | 1/2 cup | 125 mL |
| Garlic clove, minced | 1 | 1 |
| (or 1/4 tsp., 1 mL, powder) | | |
| Can of red kidney beans, | 14 oz. | 398 mL |
| rinsed and drained | | |
| Low-sodium prepared beef broth | 1/4 cup | 60 mL |
| Plain yogurt | 1/2 cup | 125 mL |
| Chopped fresh dill | 1 tbsp. | 15 mL |
| (or 3/4 tsp., 4 mL, dried) | | |
| Whole-wheat flour tortillas | 4 | 4 |
| (9 inch, 22 cm, diameter) | | |
| Chopped English cucumber | 3/4 cup | 175 mL |
| Chopped tomato | 3/4 cup | 175 mL |
| Crumbled light feta cheese (optional) | 1/4 cup | 60 mL |

Heat canola oil in large frying pan on medium-high. Add next 3 ingredients. Scramble-fry for about 8 minutes until beef is no longer pink and onion is softened.

Mash half of beans with fork on small plate. Add to beef mixture. Add remaining beans and broth. Heat and stir until hot. Remove from heat.

Combine yogurt and dill in small bowl. Spread on tortillas, almost to edge. Spoon beef mixture down centre of tortillas.

Sprinkle with remaining 3 ingredients. Fold bottom ends of tortillas over filling. Fold in sides, leaving top ends open. Makes 4 wraps.

*1 wrap: 462 Calories; 10.4 g Total Fat (3.8 g Mono, 1.6 g Poly, 3.2 g Sat); 68 mg Cholesterol; 64 g Carbohydrate; 14 g Fibre; 39 g Protein; 521 mg Sodium*

# Spicy Orange Chicken Fingers

*Familiar, family-friendly chicken fingers. Fun for the kids but with a complexity of flavours that will woo the adults. We suggest you forgo dip and eat these tasty tidbits as is.*

| | | |
|---|---|---|
| Boneless, skinless chicken breast halves (4 – 6 oz., 113 – 170 g, each) | 6 | 6 |
| Plain yogurt | 1/4 cup | 60 mL |
| Grated orange zest | 1/2 tsp. | 2 mL |
| Fine dry bread crumbs | 3/4 cup | 175 mL |
| Brown sugar, packed | 1 tbsp. | 15 mL |
| Chili powder | 1 tsp. | 5 mL |
| Ground cumin | 1/2 tsp. | 2 mL |
| Seasoned salt | 1/4 tsp. | 1 mL |
| Cayenne pepper | 1/8 tsp. | 0.5 mL |

Preheat oven to 425°F (220°C). Slice each chicken breast lengthwise into 4 strips. Combine yogurt and orange zest in large shallow bowl. Add chicken. Stir until coated.

Combine remaining 6 ingredients in large resealable freezer bag. Add half of chicken. Toss well. Arrange chicken strips in single layer on large greased baking sheet with sides. Repeat with remaining chicken and crumbs. Discard any remaining crumb mixture. Bake for about 15 minutes until chicken is no longer pink inside. Makes 24 chicken fingers. Serves 6.

*1 serving: 197 Calories; 3.0 g Total Fat (0.9 g Mono, 0.6 g Poly, 0.9 g Sat); 67 mg Cholesterol; 13 g Carbohydrate; trace Fibre; 28 g Protein; 235 mg Sodium*

---

### Paré Pointer

*For fun, chicken families go on peck-nics.*

# Orange Chicken Stir-Fry

*Orange you glad we came up with this recipe? One bite and you will be! Sweet orange and tangy mustard combine in this citrusy stir-fry. Serve over brown rice.*

| | | |
|---|---|---|
| Low-sodium prepared chicken broth | 3/4 cup | 175 mL |
| Liquid honey | 2 tbsp. | 30 mL |
| Dijon mustard | 2 tbsp. | 30 mL |
| Cornstarch | 2 tsp. | 10 mL |
| White vinegar | 1 tsp. | 5 mL |
| Grated orange zest | 1/2 tsp. | 2 mL |
| Canola oil | 1 tsp. | 5 mL |
| Boneless, skinless chicken breast halves, cut into 1/4 inch (6 mm) slices | 3/4 lb. | 340 g |
| Canola oil | 1 tsp. | 5 mL |
| Thinly sliced onion | 1/2 cup | 125 mL |
| Broccoli slaw (or shredded cabbage with carrot) | 4 1/2 cups | 1.1 L |
| Chopped broccoli | 2 cups | 500 mL |
| Can of mandarin orange segments, drained | 10 oz. | 284 mL |

Combine first 6 ingredients in small bowl. Set aside.

Heat wok or large frying pan on medium-high until very hot. Add first amount of canola oil. Add chicken. Stir-fry for about 3 minutes until no longer pink inside. Remove to plate. Set aside.

Add second amount of canola oil to hot wok. Add onion. Stir-fry for 1 to 2 minutes until onion is tender-crisp.

Add broccoli slaw, broccoli and chicken. Stir-fry for 3 to 4 minutes until broccoli is tender-crisp. Stir broth mixture. Add to wok. Heat and stir for 1 to 2 minutes until sauce is boiling and thickened. Remove from heat.

Add mandarin oranges. Toss gently. Serves 4.

*1 serving: 224 Calories; 4.2 g Total Fat (1.8 g Mono, 1.2 g Poly, 0.6 g Sat); 49 mg Cholesterol; 25 g Carbohydrate; 4 g Fibre; 23 g Protein; 197 mg Sodium*

Pictured on page 90.

# Polynesian Apricot Chicken

*Multi-tasking makes quick work of this suppertime favourite—chop the veggies while the chicken is cooking. Sweet and savoury flavours combine with just a touch of heat. Serve over rice for a complete meal.*

| | | |
|---|---|---|
| Dried apricots, quartered | 3/4 cup | 175 mL |
| Olive oil | 1 tbsp. | 15 mL |
| Boneless, skinless chicken thighs, quartered | 1 lb. | 454 g |
| Chopped onion | 1 1/2 cups | 375 mL |
| Chopped green pepper | 1 cup | 250 mL |
| Garlic clove, minced | 1 | 1 |
| (or 1/4 tsp., 1 mL, powder) | | |
| Finely grated ginger root | 1 tsp. | 5 mL |
| (or 1/4 tsp., 1 mL, ground ginger) | | |
| Chili powder | 1/2 tsp. | 2 mL |
| Ground cumin | 1/2 tsp. | 2 mL |
| Can of diced tomatoes (with juice) | 14 oz. | 398 mL |

Put apricot into small heatproof bowl. Cover with boiling water. Stir. Cover. Set aside.

Heat olive oil in large frying pan on medium. Add chicken. Cook for 8 to 10 minutes, stirring occasionally, until lightly browned. Transfer to plate. Cover to keep warm.

Add next 6 ingredients to same frying pan. Stir. Cook, covered, for about 5 minutes, stirring occasionally, until green pepper is tender-crisp.

Drain apricot. Add to green pepper mixture. Add chicken and tomatoes with juice. Stir. Increase heat to medium-high. Boil gently, uncovered, for about 10 minutes until sauce is slightly thickened. Serves 4.

*1 serving: 308 Calories; 12.1 g Total Fat (5.8 g Mono, 2.3 g Poly, 2.9 g Sat); 74 mg Cholesterol; 29 g Carbohydrate; 3 g Fibre; 23 g Protein; 363 mg Sodium*

Pictured on page 89.

# Orange-Sauced Chicken

*It's time to get saucy! Tender strips of chicken covered in a rich orange sauce with a zippy finish. Almonds add a contrasting crunch. Up the heat factor by adding more fresh chili pepper. Serve on a bed of rice.*

| | | |
|---|---|---|
| Water | 1 tbsp. | 15 mL |
| Cornstarch | 1 tsp. | 5 mL |
| Canola oil | 2 tsp. | 10 mL |
| Boneless, skinless chicken breast halves, thinly sliced | 1 lb. | 454 g |
| Paprika | 1/2 tsp. | 2 mL |
| Salt, sprinkle | | |
| Pepper, sprinkle | | |
| Orange juice | 1/4 cup | 60 mL |
| Frozen concentrated orange juice, thawed | 2 tbsp. | 30 mL |
| Grated orange zest (see Tip, page 140) | 1 tbsp. | 15 mL |
| Brown sugar, packed | 1 tsp. | 5 mL |
| Finely diced fresh hot chili pepper (see Tip, page 114), or 1/8 tsp. (0.5 mL) crushed, dried chilies | 1/2 – 1 tsp. | 2 – 5 mL |
| Sliced natural almonds | 1 – 2 tbsp. | 15 – 30 mL |

Chopped fresh parsley, for garnish

Stir water into cornstarch in small cup. Set aside.

Heat canola oil in large frying pan on medium. Add chicken. Sprinkle with next 3 ingredients. Cook for about 5 minutes, stirring often, until no longer pink inside.

Add next 5 ingredients. Stir. Bring to a boil. Stir cornstarch mixture. Add to chicken mixture. Heat and stir until boiling and thickened.

Sprinkle with almonds and parsley. Serves 4.

*1 serving: 186 Calories; 5.0 g Total Fat (2.3 g Mono, 1.3 g Poly, 0.7 g Sat); 66 mg Cholesterol; 8 g Carbohydrate; trace Fibre; 26 g Protein; 64 mg Sodium*

# Cranberry-Topped Chicken

*Fire up the grill! There's no need to save the vitamin-rich cranberries for the holidays. Ruby-red, naturally thickened cranberry sauce tops lightly seasoned, grilled chicken breasts. If you would like to use fresh parsley and sage in the sauce instead of dried, add 1/2 tsp. (2 mL) of each near the end of cooking.*

| | | |
|---|---|---|
| Olive oil | 1 tsp. | 5 mL |
| Finely chopped onion | 1/4 cup | 60 mL |
| Garlic clove, minced | 1 | 1 |
| (or 1/4 tsp., 1 mL, powder) | | |
| **CRANBERRY SAUCE** | | |
| Fresh (or frozen) cranberries | 1 cup | 250 mL |
| Low-sodium prepared chicken broth | 1/4 cup | 60 mL |
| Granulated sugar | 1/4 cup | 60 mL |
| Parsley flakes | 1/8 tsp. | 0.5 mL |
| Dried sage | 1/8 tsp. | 0.5 mL |
| Salt, sprinkle | | |
| Cayenne pepper, sprinkle | | |
| Boneless, skinless chicken breast halves | 4 | 4 |
| (4 – 6 oz., 113 – 170 g, each) | | |
| Seasoned salt, sprinkle | | |
| Pepper, sprinkle | | |

Preheat gas barbecue to medium (see Note). Heat olive oil in small frying pan on medium. Add onion and garlic. Cook for about 5 minutes, stirring occasionally, until onion is softened.

**Cranberry Sauce:** Add all 7 ingredients. Stir. Bring to a boil. Boil, uncovered, for about 5 minutes, stirring occasionally, until cranberries split and sauce is slightly thickened. Remove from heat. Cover to keep warm.

Sprinkle chicken with seasoned salt and pepper. Cook on greased grill for about 5 minutes per side until no longer pink inside. Transfer to plate. Spoon sauce over chicken. Serves 4.

*1 serving: 202 Calories; 3.1 g Total Fat (1.3 g Mono, 0.5 g Poly, 0.7 g Sat); 66 mg Cholesterol; 17 g Carbohydrate; 1 g Fibre; 26 g Protein; 66 mg Sodium*

Pictured on page 54.

**Note:** Too cold to barbecue? Chicken can be placed on a greased broiling pan and broiled on top rack in oven for about 5 minutes per side until no longer pink inside.

# Southwestern Turkey Chili

*This turkey's gone south of the border! A nice change from your regular chili.*
*Serve Sloppy Joe-style on whole-wheat buns or make it a taco salad with*
*shredded lettuce and baked whole-wheat tortilla wedges.*

| | | |
|---|---|---|
| Canola oil | 2 tsp. | 10 mL |
| Chopped onion | 1 cup | 250 mL |
| Garlic clove, minced | 1 | 1 |
| (or 1/4 tsp., 1 mL, powder) | | |
| Extra-lean ground turkey | 1 lb. | 454 g |
| Salt, sprinkle | | |
| Chopped green pepper | 1/2 cup | 125 mL |
| Chili powder | 2 tsp. | 10 mL |
| Ground cumin | 1 tsp. | 5 mL |
| Dried oregano | 1/2 tsp. | 2 mL |
| Dried crushed chilies (optional) | 1/4 tsp. | 1 mL |
| Can of black beans, rinsed and drained | 19 oz. | 540 mL |
| Low-sodium vegetable cocktail juice | 2 cups | 500 mL |
| Tomato paste (see Tip, below) | 2 tbsp. | 30 mL |
| Ketchup | 2 tbsp. | 30 mL |

Heat canola oil in large frying pan on medium-high. Add next 3 ingredients. Sprinkle with salt. Scramble-fry for about 5 minutes until onion is softened and turkey is starting to brown.

Add next 5 ingredients. Heat and stir for 1 minute.

Add remaining 4 ingredients. Stir well. Bring to a boil. Reduce heat to medium. Boil gently, uncovered, for 5 minutes, stirring occasionally, to blend flavours. Makes about 6 cups (1.5 L).

*1 cup (250 mL): 259 Calories; 3.3 g Total Fat (1.0 g Mono, 0.8 g Poly, 0.3 g Sat); 30 mg Cholesterol; 32 g Carbohydrate; 8 g Fibre; 28 g Protein; 379 mg Sodium*

 *tip*     If a recipe calls for less than an entire can of tomato paste, freeze the unopened can for 30 minutes. Open both ends and push the contents through one end. Slice off only what you need. Freeze the remaining paste in a resealable freezer bag or plastic wrap for future use.

# Mushroom Wine Chicken

*The soft and subtle sauce makes this a perfect choice for a more delicate palate. Perfect on a winter's night.*

| | | |
|---|---|---|
| Skinless, boneless chicken breast halves (4 – 6 oz., 113 – 170 g, each) | 4 | 4 |
| Olive oil | 1 tbsp. | 15 mL |
| Salt, sprinkle | | |
| Pepper | 1/4 tsp. | 1 mL |
| Sliced fresh white mushrooms | 2 cups | 500 mL |
| Garlic cloves, minced (or 1/2 tsp., 2 mL, powder) | 2 | 2 |
| All-purpose flour | 2 tbsp. | 30 mL |
| Low-sodium prepared chicken broth | 1 cup | 250 mL |
| Dry (or alcohol-free) red wine | 1/2 cup | 125 mL |
| Dried thyme | 1/2 tsp. | 2 mL |

Place chicken breasts between 2 sheets of plastic wrap. Pound with mallet or rolling pin to about 1/2 inch (12 mm) thickness.

Heat olive oil in large frying pan on medium-high. Add chicken. Sprinkle with salt and pepper. Cook for about 3 minutes per side until lightly browned. Transfer to plate. Cover to keep warm.

Add mushrooms and garlic to same frying pan. Cook on medium for about 3 minutes, stirring occasionally, until softened and starting to brown.

Add flour. Heat and stir for 1 minute. Slowly add broth and wine, stirring constantly. Add thyme. Heat and stir until boiling and thickened. Add chicken. Reduce heat to medium-low. Simmer, uncovered, for 5 minutes to blend flavours. Serves 4.

*1 serving: 212 Calories; 5.6 g Total Fat (3.0 g Mono, 0.8 g Poly, 1.0 g Sat); 66 mg Cholesterol; 6 g Carbohydrate; 1 g Fibre; 28 g Protein; 75 mg Sodium*

 Don't keep this good news in the dark—mushrooms are a good source of vitamins B2, B3 and B5. Vitamin B2 is also called riboflavin and aids in the breakdown of carbohydrates, fats and proteins. Vitamin B3 is also known as niacin and aids in the upkeep of healthy skin and nerves. Vitamin B5, also called pantothenic acid, is essential in proper cell metabolism.

# Sweet-And-Sour Chicken

*With the flavourful combination of mustard, lime and pineapple, this is not your everyday chicken dish! We've made sure there's plenty of sauce for you to serve over egg noodles or rice.*

| | | |
|---|---|---|
| Pineapple juice | 1/4 cup | 60 mL |
| Brown sugar, packed | 3 tbsp. | 50 mL |
| Balsamic vinegar | 2 tbsp. | 30 mL |
| Dijon mustard | 2 tbsp. | 30 mL |
| Lime juice | 2 tbsp. | 30 mL |
| Cornstarch | 2 tsp. | 10 mL |
| Canola oil | 2 tsp. | 10 mL |
| Boneless, skinless chicken breast halves, cut into 1 inch (2.5 cm) cubes | 1 lb. | 454 g |
| Canola oil | 2 tsp. | 10 mL |
| Chopped red pepper | 1 cup | 250 mL |
| Chopped onion | 1/2 cup | 125 mL |
| Garlic clove, minced (or 1/4 tsp., 1 mL, powder) | 1 | 1 |

Combine first 6 ingredients in small bowl. Set aside.

Heat wok or large frying pan on medium-high until very hot. Add first amount of canola oil. Add chicken. Stir-fry for about 4 minutes until browned. Transfer to plate.

Add second amount of canola oil to hot wok. Add next 3 ingredients. Stir-fry for about 2 minutes until onion is softened. Add chicken. Stir pineapple juice mixture. Add to chicken mixture. Heat and stir for about 1 minute until sauce is boiling and thickened. Serves 4.

*1 serving: 242 Calories; 6.5 g Total Fat (3.1 g Mono, 1.8 g Poly, 0.8 g Sat); 66 mg Cholesterol; 19 g Carbohydrate; 1 g Fibre; 26 g Protein; 169 mg Sodium*

# Grilled Pepper Chicken

*Add flair to your food the easiest way possible—with rustic grill marks!*
*Balsamic vinegar and feta cheese add delicious flavour to colourful sweet*
*peppers and tender chicken.*

| | | |
|---|---|---|
| Boneless, skinless chicken breast halves<br>(4 – 6 oz., 113 g – 170 g, each) | 4 | 4 |
| Salt, sprinkle | | |
| Pepper, sprinkle | | |
| Small red pepper, quartered lengthwise | 1 | 1 |
| Small orange pepper, quartered lengthwise | 1 | 1 |
| Small yellow pepper, quartered lengthwise | 1 | 1 |
| Olive oil | 1 tbsp. | 15 mL |
| Ground oregano | 1/2 tsp. | 2 mL |
| Pepper, sprinkle | | |
| Balsamic vinegar | 2 tbsp. | 30 mL |
| Crumbled light feta cheese | 1/4 cup | 60 mL |
| Finely chopped fresh parsley | 2 tsp. | 10 mL |

Preheat gas barbecue to medium-high (see Note). Sprinkle chicken with salt and pepper. Cook on greased grill for about 3 minutes per side until no longer pink inside.

Meanwhile, put next 3 ingredients into large bowl. Drizzle with olive oil. Sprinkle with oregano and pepper. Toss well. Cook on grill for about 3 minutes per side until tender-crisp.

Transfer chicken and peppers to large bowl. Drizzle with balsamic vinegar. Toss. Transfer to large plate.

Sprinkle with feta and parsley. Serves 4.

*1 serving:* *196 Calories; 6.5 g Total Fat (3.0 g Mono, 0.8 g Poly, 1.7 g Sat); 68 mg Cholesterol;*
*6 g Carbohydrate; 1 g Fibre; 28 g Protein; 201 mg Sodium*

Pictured on page 125.

**Note:** Too cold to barbecue? Chicken and peppers can be placed on a greased broiling pan and broiled on top rack in oven for about 5 minutes per side until chicken is no longer pink inside.

# Mango Salsa Chicken

*Refreshing, delicious and pretty to look at! Spicy citrus and mango salsa is the perfect match for tender chicken. The salsa also goes well with salads, wraps, quesadillas and grilled fish.*

| | | |
|---|---|---|
| Boneless, skinless chicken breast halves (4 – 6 oz., 113 g – 170 g, each) | 4 | 4 |
| Olive oil | 2 tbsp. | 30 mL |
| Lime juice | 1 1/2 tbsp. | 25 mL |
| Grated lime zest | 1 1/2 tsp. | 7 mL |
| Cajun seasoning | 1 tsp. | 5 mL |
| **LIME MANGO SALSA** | | |
| Chopped frozen mango, thawed (see Note) | 1 cup | 250 mL |
| Finely diced red onion | 1/4 cup | 60 mL |
| Garlic clove, minced (or 1/4 tsp., 1 mL, powder) | 1 | 1 |
| Finely diced jalapeño pepper (see Tip, page 114) | 2 tbsp. | 30 mL |
| Olive oil | 2 tbsp. | 30 mL |
| Lime juice | 1 1/2 tbsp. | 25 mL |
| Chopped fresh cilantro or parsley | 1 tbsp. | 15 mL |
| Grated lime zest | 1 1/2 tsp. | 7 mL |

Preheat gas barbecue to medium (see Note). Score both sides of each chicken breast several times with sharp knife. Combine next 4 ingredients in small bowl. Brush over chicken breasts. Cook chicken on greased grill for about 6 minutes per side, brushing with lime mixture, until no longer pink inside.

**Lime Mango Salsa:** Combine all 8 ingredients in small bowl. Makes 1 1/2 cups (375 mL) salsa. Serve with chicken. Serves 4.

*1 serving: 281 Calories; 15.5 g Total Fat (10.5 g Mono, 1.6 g Poly, 2.3 g Sat); 65 mg Cholesterol; 10 g Carbohydrate; 1 g Fibre; 26 g Protein; 197 mg Sodium*

Pictured on page 89.

**Note:** If frozen mango is unavailable, fresh or canned mango can be used instead.

**Note:** Too cold to barbecue? Chicken can be placed on a greased broiling pan and broiled on top rack in oven for about 5 minutes per side until no longer pink inside.

**Variation:** Use chopped oranges or pineapple instead of mango.

# Dill Turkey Burgers

*So, you say you're a dill pickle lover? Don't just garnish your burger with pickles, cook them right in for a more intense flavour. Garnish with your favourite fixings.*

| | | |
|---|---|---|
| Large egg, fork-beaten | 1 | 1 |
| Whole-wheat bread slices, processed into crumbs (about 3/4 cup, 175 mL) | 2 | 2 |
| Finely chopped dill pickle | 1/4 cup | 60 mL |
| Chopped fresh dill (or 1/2 tsp., 2 mL, dried) | 2 tsp. | 10 mL |
| Lemon pepper | 1 tsp. | 5 mL |
| Extra-lean ground turkey | 1 lb. | 454 g |
| Olive oil | 1 tbsp. | 15 mL |
| Prepared mustard | 2 tsp. | 10 mL |
| Whole-wheat hamburger buns, split | 4 | 4 |
| Large tomato, thinly sliced | 1 | 1 |

Combine first 5 ingredients in medium bowl. Add turkey. Mix well. Divide into 4 equal portions. Shape into 1/2 inch (12 mm) thick patties.

Heat olive oil in large frying pan on medium. Add patties. Cook for about 7 minutes per side until fully cooked, and internal temperature of turkey reaches 175°F (80°C).

Spread mustard on bottom halves of buns. Serve patties, topped with tomato slices, in buns. Makes 4 burgers.

*1 burger: 327 Calories; 8.9 g Total Fat (3.8 g Mono, 1.6 g Poly, 1.3 g Sat); 92 mg Cholesterol; 31 g Carbohydrate; 5 g Fibre; 35 g Protein; 586 mg Sodium*

1. Polynesian Apricot Chicken, page 80
2. Mango Salsa Chicken, page 87

Props courtesy of: Dansk Gifts
Mikasa Home Store

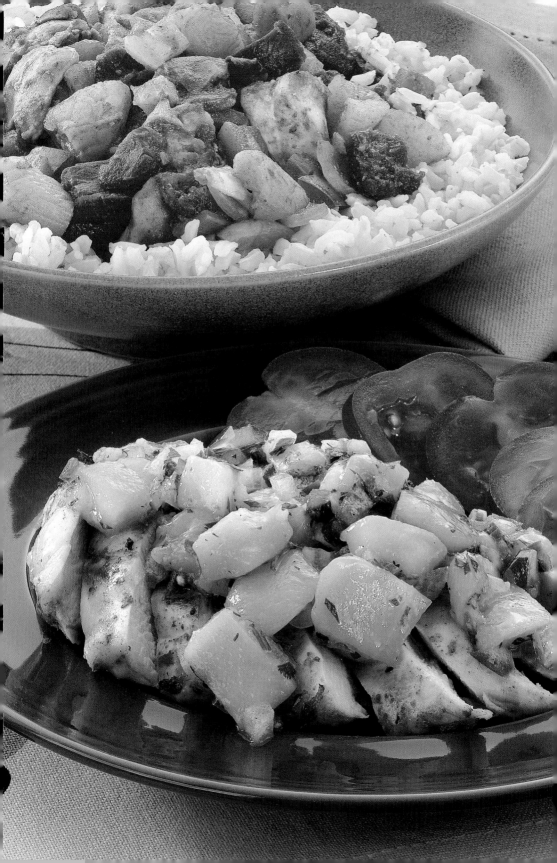

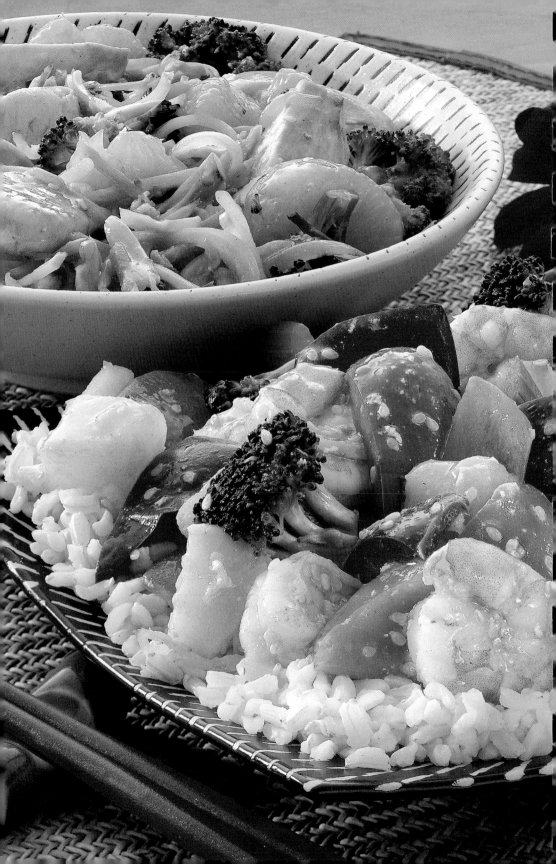

# Tarragon-Poached Fish

*Silky tarragon and lemon sauce is the perfect match for fish. There will be lots of sauce to serve over rice or noodles. Simply delicious!*

| | | |
|---|---|---|
| Butter (or hard margarine) | 2 tbsp. | 30 mL |
| All-purpose flour | 2 tbsp. | 30 mL |
| Prepared vegetable broth | 1 cup | 250 mL |
| Lemon juice | 2 tbsp. | 30 mL |
| Dried tarragon | 1 tsp. | 5 mL |
| Fresh (or frozen, thawed) haddock (or cod) fillets (about 1/2 inch, 12 mm, thick), any small bones removed | 1 lb. | 454 g |
| Chopped fresh tarragon, for garnish | | |

Melt butter in large frying pan on medium. Sprinkle with flour. Heat and stir for 1 minute. Slowly add broth, stirring constantly, until boiling and thickened.

Add lemon juice and tarragon. Stir.

Pat fillets dry with paper towels. Add to sauce. Reduce heat to medium-low. Simmer, covered, for 5 to 7 minutes until fish flakes easily when tested with fork.

Garnish with tarragon. Serves 4.

*1 serving: 168 Calories; 6.6 g Total Fat (1.6 g Mono, 0.5 g Poly, 3.8 g Sat); 80 mg Cholesterol; 4 g Carbohydrate; trace Fibre; 22 g Protein; 235 mg Sodium*

Pictured on page 143.

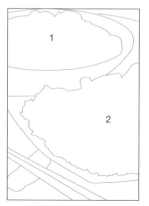

1. Orange Chicken Stir-Fry, page 79
2. Aloha Shrimp Stir-Fry, page 92

Props courtesy of: Dansk Gifts
Linens 'N Things

# Aloha Shrimp Stir-Fry

*Mahalo nui loa—or thank you very much! Your dinner guests will certainly thank you for bringing this tropical taste to the table! Colourful fresh vegetables and shrimp with a sweet pineapple-ginger glaze. Enjoy with a Mai Tai!*

| | | |
|---|---|---|
| Low-sodium prepared chicken broth | 1/2 cup | 125 mL |
| Reserved pineapple juice | 2 tbsp. | 30 mL |
| Low-sodium soy sauce | 2 tsp. | 10 mL |
| Cornstarch | 2 tsp. | 10 mL |
| Chili paste (sambal oelek) | 1/2 tsp. | 2 mL |
| Canola oil | 2 tsp. | 10 mL |
| Frozen uncooked large shrimp (peeled and deveined), thawed | 1 lb. | 454 g |
| Garlic clove, minced (or 1/4 tsp., 1 mL, powder) | 1 | 1 |
| Finely grated ginger root (or 1/8 tsp., 0.5 mL, ground ginger) | 1/2 tsp. | 2 mL |
| Canola oil | 2 tsp. | 10 mL |
| Fresh mixed stir-fry vegetables | 5 cups | 1.25 L |
| Can of pineapple chunks, drained and juice reserved | 19 oz. | 540 mL |
| Sesame seeds, toasted (see Tip, page 14), optional | 1 tbsp. | 15 mL |

Stir first 5 ingredients in small cup until smooth. Set aside.

Heat wok or large frying pan on medium-high until very hot. Add first amount of canola oil. Add next 3 ingredients. Stir-fry for about 2 minutes until shrimp turn pink. Transfer to small bowl.

Heat second amount of canola oil in same wok. Add vegetables. Stir-fry for about 3 minutes until tender-crisp. Add pineapple and shrimp. Toss. Stir broth mixture. Add to vegetable mixture. Heat and stir for about 1 minute until boiling and slightly thickened.

Sprinkle with sesame seeds. Serves 6.

*1 serving: 179 Calories; 4.5 g Total Fat (2.0 g Mono, 1.5 g Poly, 0.5 g Sat); 115 mg Cholesterol; 18 g Carbohydrate; 2 g Fibre; 17 g Protein; 194 mg Sodium*

Pictured on page 90.

# Honey Ginger Salmon

*Keep your honey happy and healthy with this delicious and attractive combination! A light, sweet glaze complements salmon garnished with crunchy cucumber salsa—a refreshing choice for supper on a warm summer evening.*

| | | |
|---|---|---|
| Fresh (or frozen, thawed) salmon fillets (about 1 lb., 454 g), skin removed | 4 | 4 |
| Liquid honey | 1/4 cup | 60 mL |
| Rice vinegar | 2 tbsp. | 30 mL |
| Finely grated ginger root (or 1/4 tsp., 1 mL, ground ginger) | 1 tsp. | 5 mL |
| **CUCUMBER SALSA** | | |
| Diced English cucumber | 1 cup | 250 mL |
| Chopped green onion | 1/4 cup | 60 mL |
| Diced yellow pepper | 1/4 cup | 60 mL |
| Liquid honey | 1 tbsp. | 15 mL |
| Rice vinegar | 1 tbsp. | 15 mL |
| Salt | 1/2 tsp. | 2 mL |
| Pepper | 1/4 tsp. | 1 mL |

Preheat broiler. Arrange fillets on greased baking sheet with sides. Combine next 3 ingredients in small cup. Brush generously over fillets. Broil on centre rack in oven for 8 to 10 minutes until fish flakes easily when tested with fork.

**Cucumber Salsa:** Meanwhile, combine all 7 ingredients in small bowl. Makes about 1 1/4 cups (300 mL) salsa. Serve with salmon. Serves 4.

*1 serving: 303 Calories; 12.4 g Total Fat (4.4 g Mono, 4.5 g Poly, 2.5 g Sat); 67 mg Cholesterol; 24 g Carbohydrate; 1 g Fibre; 23 g Protein; 363 mg Sodium*

Pictured on front cover.

 Hook, line and sinker, fish is a great source of lean protein and omega-3 fatty acids, which aid in preventing build-up from forming in your arteries. Truly a heart-friendly food.

# Corn And Cod Tacos

*A nice light change from heavier ground beef and cheese-filled tacos. Add chopped avocado to the salsa for a nutrient booster. To save time, set out the lettuce, fish, salsa and taco shells so everyone can build their own.*

| | | |
|---|---|---|
| Fresh (or frozen, thawed) cod fillets, any small bones removed | 1 lb. | 454 g |
| Lime juice | 1 tbsp. | 15 mL |
| Ground cumin | 1 tsp. | 5 mL |
| Hard taco shells | 8 | 8 |
| CORN SALSA | | |
| Frozen kernel corn, thawed (see Tip, page 67) | 1 cup | 250 mL |
| Medium salsa | 1/2 cup | 125 mL |
| Chopped fresh cilantro | 1/4 cup | 60 mL |
| Shredded lettuce, lightly packed | 1 cup | 250 mL |

Preheat broiler. Arrange fillets in single layer on greased baking sheet with sides. Drizzle with lime juice. Sprinkle with cumin. Broil on centre rack in oven for 8 to 10 minutes until fish flakes easily when tested with fork. Break into small chunks. Set aside.

Arrange taco shells in single layer on separate ungreased baking sheet. Place on bottom rack in hot oven for 1 minute until warm.

**Corn Salsa:** Meanwhile, combine all 4 ingredients in small bowl. Makes about 1 cup (250 mL) salsa.

Layer lettuce, fish and Corn Salsa, in order given, in taco shells. Makes 8 tacos.

*1 taco: 134 Calories; 3.5 g Total Fat (1.3 g Mono, 1.3 g Poly, 0.5 g Sat); 21 mg Cholesterol; 14 g Carbohydrate; 2 g Fibre; 12 g Protein; 155 mg Sodium*

Pictured on page 72.

# Oven-Poached Salmon Steaks

*Simple can be so good! Very mildly flavoured salmon with the perfect complement—a light dill sauce. Wonderful served with a vegetable salad and rice pilaf.*

| | | |
|---|---|---|
| Water | 1 1/2 cups | 375 mL |
| Chopped onion | 1/4 cup | 60 mL |
| Lemon juice | 2 tbsp. | 30 mL |
| Bay leaf, broken in half | 1 | 1 |
| Fresh (or frozen, thawed) salmon steaks (4 – 5 oz., 113 – 140 g, each), about 1 inch (2.5 cm) thick | 4 | 4 |
| Pepper, sprinkle | | |
| Plain yogurt | 1/2 cup | 125 mL |
| Chopped fresh dill | 1/4 cup | 60 mL |
| Dijon mustard | 2 tsp. | 10 mL |
| Worcestershire sauce | 1/4 tsp. | 1 mL |

Preheat oven to 325°F (160°C). Combine first 4 ingredients in 2 cup (500 mL) liquid measure or small microwave-safe bowl. Microwave on high (100%) until boiling. Pour half of water mixture into 2 quart (2 L) shallow baking dish.

Arrange salmon in single layer in baking dish. Sprinkle with pepper. Pour remaining water mixture over salmon. Bake for about 15 minutes until fish flakes easily when tested with fork. Transfer to serving plate. Discard bay leaf and poaching liquid.

Meanwhile, combine remaining 4 ingredients in small cup. Serve with salmon. Serves 4.

*1 serving: 233 Calories; 13.3 g Total Fat (4.7 g Mono, 4.5 g Poly, 3.1 g Sat); 71 mg Cholesterol; 3 g Carbohydrate; trace Fibre; 24 g Protein; 117 mg Sodium*

 *fyi* Look for yogurts that contain live and active bacterial culture. Studies have shown that these "good" bacteria may help maintain a healthy digestive tract.

# Seafood Medley

*Ahoy, me hearties! This light stew is perfect for anyone who's angling for a dinner from the high seas! Morsels of seafood in a tomato sauce—reminiscent of cioppino. Serve over rice or pasta.*

| | | |
|---|---|---|
| Canola (or olive) oil | 2 tsp. | 10 mL |
| Finely chopped onion | 1/2 cup | 125 mL |
| Garlic cloves, minced | 2 | 2 |
| Can of diced tomatoes (with juice) | 14 oz. | 398 mL |
| Low-sodium prepared chicken broth | 1/2 cup | 125 mL |
| Grated lemon zest | 1 tbsp. | 15 mL |
| Ground cumin | 1/2 tsp. | 2 mL |
| Pepper | 1/8 tsp. | 0.5 mL |
| Chopped capers (optional) | 1 tbsp. | 15 mL |
| Fresh (or frozen, thawed) salmon fillet, skin removed, cut into 1 inch (2.5 cm) pieces | 6 oz. | 170 g |
| Fresh (or frozen, thawed) halibut fillet, any small bones removed, cut into 1 inch (2.5 cm) pieces | 6 oz. | 170 g |
| Fresh (or frozen, thawed) large sea scallops, halved | 1/4 lb. | 113 g |
| Chopped fresh parsley | 1/4 cup | 60 mL |

Heat canola oil in large frying pan on medium-high. Add onion and garlic. Cook for about 5 minutes, stirring occasionally, until onion is softened.

Add next 6 ingredients. Stir. Cook, covered, for 3 minutes, stirring occasionally, to blend flavours.

Add remaining 4 ingredients. Stir. Reduce heat to medium-low. Simmer, covered, for about 4 minutes until fish flakes easily when tested with fork and scallops are opaque. Makes about 4 cups (1 L).

*1 cup (250 mL): 203 Calories; 8.3 g Total Fat (3.4 g Mono, 2.8 g Poly, 1.3 g Sat); 48 mg Cholesterol; 8 g Carbohydrate; 1 g Fibre; 24 g Protein; 372 mg Sodium*

# Sesame Ginger Halibut

*Light flavours with an Asian twist and an upscale presentation. Snowy white halibut glazed with sesame, ginger and pepper is served alongside tender-crisp, ginger-infused bok choy.*

| | | |
|---|---|---|
| Sesame oil | 2 tsp. | 10 mL |
| Water | 1 cup | 250 mL |
| Prepared vegetable broth | 1/2 cup | 125 mL |
| Chopped green onion | 1/2 cup | 125 mL |
| Finely grated gingerroot | 1 tbsp. | 15 mL |
| Chopped bok choy | 4 cups | 1 L |
| Fresh (or frozen, thawed) halibut fillets (4 – 5 oz., 113 – 140 g each), any small bones removed | 4 | 4 |
| Pepper | 1/4 tsp. | 1 mL |
| Tahini (sesame paste) | 1 tbsp. | 15 mL |
| Rice vinegar | 1 tbsp. | 15 mL |
| Low-sodium soy sauce | 2 tsp. | 10 mL |
| Sesame oil | 1/2 tsp. | 2 mL |
| Sesame seeds, toasted (see Tip, page 14) | 2 tsp. | 10 mL |

Heat sesame oil in large frying pan on medium-high. Add next 4 ingredients. Bring to a boil. Add bok choy.

Place fillets over bok choy. Sprinkle with pepper. Reduce heat to medium-low. Simmer, covered, for about 3 minutes until bok choy starts to soften.

Combine next 4 ingredients in small cup. Drizzle over fillets. Cook, covered, for about 5 minutes until fish flakes easily when tested with fork. Transfer fillets and bok choy to serving plate, using slotted spoon.  Drizzle sauce over top.

Sprinkle with sesame seeds. Serves 4.

*1 serving: 184 Calories; 6.9 g Total Fat (2.5 g Mono, 2.7 g Poly, 1.0 g Sat); 36 mg Cholesterol; 4 g Carbohydrate; 1 g Fibre; 25 g Protein; 312 mg Sodium*

# Graham-Crusted Basa

*A tantalizing taste surprise! A sweet coating of graham crumbs and crunchy nuts over moist, delicate fish. Just a hint of lemon rounds out this delicious dish.*

| | | |
|---|---|---|
| Graham cracker crumbs | 1/2 cup | 125 mL |
| Finely chopped pecans | 2 tbsp. | 30 mL |
| Grated lemon zest | 1 tsp. | 5 mL |
| Lemon pepper | 1/4 tsp. | 1 mL |
| Milk | 1/4 cup | 60 mL |
| Fresh (or frozen, thawed) basa (or other white fish) fillets (4 – 5 oz., 113 – 140 g, each), any small bones removed | 4 | 4 |
| Cooking spray | | |

Preheat oven to 400°F (205°C). Combine first 4 ingredients in shallow bowl.

Measure milk into separate shallow bowl.

Dip fillets into milk. Press both sides of fillets into crumb mixture until coated. Place fillets on greased baking sheet with sides. Discard any remaining milk and crumbs. Spray fillets lightly with cooking spray. Bake for about 10 minutes until fish flakes easily when tested with fork. Serves 4.

*1 serving: 229 Calories; 10.5 g Total Fat (4.2 g Mono, 3.6 g Poly, 1.5 g Sat); 69 mg Cholesterol; 9 g Carbohydrate; 1 g Fibre; 23 g Protein; 135 mg Sodium*

# Lemon Sole

*You won't be standing on your feet for long—this lemony, breaded sole dish is easy on the soles, not to mention good for the soul! Assembles and bakes quickly.*

| | | |
|---|---|---|
| Fine dry bread crumbs | 1 cup | 250 mL |
| Grated zest from 1 small lemon | | |
| Salt, sprinkle | | |
| Pepper, sprinkle | | |
| Large egg | 1 | 1 |
| Fresh (or frozen, thawed) sole fillets (4 – 5 oz., 113 – 140 g, each), any small bones removed | 6 | 6 |

*(continued on next page)*

Fish & Seafood

Preheat oven to 400°F (205°C). Combine first 4 ingredients in shallow bowl.

Beat egg in separate shallow bowl.

Dip fillets into egg. Press both sides of fillets into crumb mixture until coated. Place on greased baking sheet with sides. Bake for about 5 minutes until fish flakes easily when tested with fork. Serves 6.

*1 serving: 187 Calories; 3.2 g Total Fat (1.1 g Mono, 0.7 g Poly, 0.8 g Sat); 85 mg Cholesterol; 13 g Carbohydrate; trace Fibre; 25 g Protein; 257 mg Sodium*

---

# Halibut Bake

*A slightly sweet, creamy spread hides beneath a crispy crumb coating. A dashing dash of dill adds the perfect touch.*

| | | |
|---|---|---|
| **Fresh (or frozen, thawed) halibut fillets (4 – 5 oz., 113 – 140 g, each), any small bones removed** | 4 | 4 |
| **Sweet pickle relish** | 1/4 cup | 60 mL |
| **Light mayonnaise** | 2 tbsp. | 30 mL |
| **Grated Parmesan cheese** | 2 tbsp. | 30 mL |
| **Creamed horseradish** | 1 tsp. | 5 mL |
| **Cornflake crumbs** | 1/4 cup | 60 mL |
| **Fine dry bread crumbs** | 1/4 cup | 60 mL |
| **Dried dillweed** | 1/2 tsp. | 2 mL |

Preheat oven to 400°F (205°C). Pat fillets dry with paper towels. Arrange in single layer in greased 3 quart (3 L) shallow baking dish.

Combine next 4 ingredients in small bowl. Spread over fillets.

Combine remaining 3 ingredients in separate small bowl. Sprinkle over fillets. Bake for about 15 minutes until fish flakes easily when tested with fork. Serves 4.

*1 serving: 418 Calories; 7.3 g Total Fat (1.6 g Mono, 1.1 g Poly, 1.5 g Sat); 42 mg Cholesterol; 66 g Carbohydrate; 2 g Fibre; 27 g Protein; 1558 mg Sodium*

# Salmon With Citrus Salsa

*Don't you love it when such a minimal effort reaps such a huge reward?
This is the type of healthy, yet decadent, meal you would expect to
get at a very posh spa. The pairing of citrus and salmon is
a delicious and refreshing combination!*

**QUICK CITRUS SALSA**

| | | |
|---|---|---|
| Large orange, segmented and chopped (see Note) | 1 | 1 |
| Small ruby red grapefruit, segmented and chopped (see Note) | 1 | 1 |
| Finely chopped red onion | 1/4 cup | 60 mL |
| Chopped fresh cilantro or parsley | 1 tsp. | 5 mL |
| Small fresh hot chili pepper, finely diced (see Tip, page 100) | 1 | 1 |
| Salt, sprinkle | | |
| Pepper, sprinkle | | |

**SALMON**

| | | |
|---|---|---|
| Fresh (or frozen, thawed) salmon fillets (about 4 – 5 oz., 113 – 140 g, each), skin removed | 4 | 4 |
| Salt, sprinkle | | |
| Pepper, sprinkle | | |

**Quick Citrus Salsa:** Combine all 7 ingredients in small bowl. Makes about 1 1/3 cups (325 mL) salsa. Set aside.

**Salmon:** Preheat broiler. Sprinkle fillets with salt and pepper. Place on greased baking sheet with sides. Broil on top rack in oven for about 5 minutes until fish flakes easily when tested with fork. Serve with Quick Citrus Salsa. Serves 4.

*1 serving: 250 Calories; 12.4 g Total Fat (4.4 g Mono, 4.5 g Poly, 2.5 g Sat); 67 mg Cholesterol; 11 g Carbohydrate; 2 g Fibre; 23 g Protein; 68 mg Sodium*

**Note:** To segment citrus fruits, trim a small slice of peel from both ends so the flesh is exposed. Place the fruit, cut-side down, on a cutting board. Remove the peel with a sharp knife, cutting down and around the flesh, leaving as little pith as possible. Over a small bowl, cut on either side of the membranes to release the segments.

Fish & Seafood

# Poached Salmon Kabobs

*Delicate salmon skewers on a bed of nutty couscous with a burst of fresh lemon. A very attractive presentation, indeed!*

| | | |
|---|---|---|
| Low-sodium prepared chicken broth | 1/2 cup | 125 mL |
| Orange juice | 1/2 cup | 125 mL |
| Olive oil | 1 tsp. | 5 mL |
| Cayenne pepper, sprinkle (optional) | | |
| Couscous | 1 cup | 250 mL |
| Low-sodium prepared chicken broth | 2 cups | 500 mL |
| Chopped onion | 1/2 cup | 125 mL |
| Garlic cloves, minced | 3 | 3 |
| (or 3/4 tsp., 4 mL, powder) | | |
| Pepper | 1 tsp. | 5 mL |
| Large lemon, cut into 8 wedges | 1 | 1 |
| Fresh (or frozen, thawed) salmon fillets, skin removed, cut into 1 inch (2.5 cm) cubes | 1 lb. | 454 g |
| Bamboo skewers (8 inches, 20 cm, each) | 4 | 4 |
| Chopped fresh dill | 1 1/2 tsp. | 7 mL |

Measure first 4 ingredients into medium saucepan. Bring to a boil. Remove from heat. Add couscous. Stir. Cover. Let stand for about 5 minutes until liquid is absorbed.

Meanwhile, combine next 4 ingredients in medium frying pan. Stir. Add 4 lemon wedges. Bring to a boil. Reduce heat to medium-low.

Thread fish onto skewers. Add to broth mixture. Simmer, covered, for about 5 minutes until fish flakes easily when tested with fork. Fluff couscous with fork. Spoon onto serving platter. Place skewers over top.

Sprinkle with dill. Serve with remaining lemon wedges. Serves 4.

*1 serving: 439 Calories; 14.4 g Total Fat (5.5 g Mono, 4.8 g Poly, 2.9 g Sat); 67 mg Cholesterol; 48 g Carbohydrate; 5 g Fibre; 31 g Protein; 97 mg Sodium*

Despair not, there are some good fats out there. Monounsaturated fats, like those in olive oil, help to reduce the levels of bad cholesterol in your body.

# Tomato Shrimp Pasta

*A garlic lover's dream come true! Tangy tomato sauce with lots of shrimp, plenty of pasta and mild chili heat to liven things up. Serve with a sprinkle of grated Parmesan and fresh ground pepper.*

| | | |
|---|---|---|
| Whole-wheat spaghetti | 8 oz. | 225 g |
| Olive oil | 2 tbsp. | 30 mL |
| Garlic cloves, minced | 3 | 3 |
| (or 3/4 tsp., 4 mL, powder) | | |
| Cans of diced tomatoes (with juice), | 2 | 2 |
| 14 oz., 398 mL, each | | |
| Dried crushed chilies | 1/2 tsp. | 2 mL |
| Frozen uncooked large shrimp | 1 lb. | 454 g |
| (peeled and deveined), thawed | | |
| Grated lemon zest | 1 tsp. | 5 mL |
| Chopped fresh parsley | 1/4 cup | 60 mL |

Cook spaghetti in boiling salted water in large uncovered saucepan or Dutch oven for about 8 minutes, stirring occasionally, until tender but firm. Drain. Return to same pot. Cover to keep warm.

Meanwhile, heat olive oil in large frying pan on medium. Add garlic. Cook for 1 minute until fragrant. Add tomatoes with juice and chilies. Stir. Boil gently for about 5 minutes until slightly thickened.

Add shrimp and lemon zest. Return to a boil. Cook and stir for about 4 minutes until shrimp turn pink. Add parsley. Stir. Add to spaghetti. Toss. Serves 4.

*1 serving: 416 Calories; 9.6 g Total Fat (5.4 g Mono, 1.7 g Poly, 1.4 g Sat); 172 mg Cholesterol; 53 g Carbohydrate; 5 g Fibre; 33 g Protein; 730 mg Sodium*

# Fennel Snapper Packets

*Good things come in small packets! Get your protein and vegetables all wrapped up in one convenient package. Perfect with a squeeze of lemon.*

| | | |
|---|---|---|
| Thinly sliced fennel bulb (white part only) | 1 cup | 250 mL |
| Thinly sliced onion | 1/4 cup | 60 mL |
| Chopped fresh parsley | 1 tbsp. | 15 mL |
| (or 3/4 tsp., 4 mL, flakes) | | |
| Olive oil | 1 tsp. | 5 mL |
| Salt, sprinkle | | |
| Pepper, sprinkle | | |
| Fresh (or frozen, thawed) snapper fillet, | 1/2 lb. | 225 g |
| any small bones removed | | |
| Dry (or alcohol-free) white wine | 2 tbsp. | 30 mL |
| Salt, sprinkle | | |
| Lemon wedges (optional) | 2 | 2 |

Preheat oven to 400°F (205°C). Combine first 3 ingredients in medium bowl. Drizzle with olive oil. Sprinkle with salt and pepper. Toss well. Divide fennel mixture on 2 sheets of greased heavy-duty (or double layer of regular) foil.

Cut fillet into 2 portions. Place over fennel mixture. Drizzle with wine. Sprinkle with salt. Fold edges of foil together over fish to enclose. Fold ends to seal completely. Place packets, seam-side up, on ungreased baking sheet with sides. Bake for 15 to 20 minutes until fish flakes easily when tested with fork.

Squeeze lemon over top. Serves 2.

*1 serving: 211 Calories; 4.2 g Total Fat (2.0 g Mono, 0.7 g Poly, 0.6 g Sat); 42 mg Cholesterol; 16 g Carbohydrate; 6 g Fibre; 26 g Protein; 171 mg Sodium*

## Paré Pointer

*When telephone wires are high up in the air,*
*they keep up conversation.*

# Ricotta Rotini

*This rich and creamy dish is a pasta and cheese lover's dream come true. Try with some basil or sun-dried tomato pesto for a more assertive flavour.*

| | | |
|---|---|---|
| Whole-wheat rotini | 5 cups | 1.25 L |
| Olive oil | 2 tsp. | 10 mL |
| Sliced red onion | 1 cup | 250 mL |
| Garlic cloves, minced | 2 | 2 |
| (or 1/2 tsp., 2 mL, powder) | | |
| All-purpose flour | 2 tbsp. | 30 mL |
| Can of evaporated milk | 13 1/2 oz. | 385 mL |
| Ricotta cheese | 1 cup | 250 mL |
| Jar of marinated artichoke hearts, | 6 oz. | 170 mL |
| drained and chopped | | |
| Cherry tomatoes, halved | 12 | 12 |
| Grated Parmesan cheese | 1/4 cup | 60 mL |
| Chopped fresh parsley | 2 tbsp. | 30 mL |
| Grated Parmesan cheese (optional) | 2 – 4 tbsp. | 30 – 60 mL |

Cook pasta in boiling salted water in large uncovered saucepan or Dutch oven for about 12 minutes, stirring occasionally, until tender but firm. Drain. Return to saucepan. Cover to keep warm.

Meanwhile, heat olive oil in large frying pan on medium. Add onion and garlic. Cook for 5 to 10 minutes, stirring occasionally, until onion is softened.

Sprinkle with flour. Heat and stir for 1 minute.

Slowly add milk, stirring constantly until mixture is boiling and thickened.

Add next 3 ingredients. Stir. Cook for about 4 minutes, stirring often, until tomato is starting to soften. Add to pasta.

Add first amount of Parmesan cheese and parsley. Stir.

Sprinkle with second amount of Parmesan cheese. Serves 4.

*1 serving: 702 Calories; 22.7 g Total Fat (6.9 g Mono, 0.8 g Poly, 22.7 g Sat); 66 mg Cholesterol; 95 g Carbohydrate; 12 g Fibre; 31 g Protein; 333 mg Sodium*

# Eggplant Envelopes

*With nary a bill in sight, you'll be delighted to open up these envelopes. Sweet little eggplant packages come bearing tasty gifts—feta cheese, pesto and roasted red pepper. Your nearest and dearest will marvel at the unique presentation.*

| | | |
|---|---|---|
| Medium eggplant (with peel), cut lengthwise into 8 1/4 inch (6 mm) thick slices | 1 | 1 |
| Basil pesto | 2 tbsp. | 30 mL |
| Crumbled light feta cheese | 3/4 cup | 175 mL |
| Roasted red peppers, drained and blotted dry, chopped | 1/2 cup | 125 mL |
| Olive oil | 1 tbsp. | 15 mL |
| Salt, sprinkle | | |
| Pepper, sprinkle | | |

Preheat oven to 450°F (230°C). Meanwhile, cook eggplant slices in boiling water in Dutch oven for about 2 minutes until softened. Remove to paper towels to drain.

Lay 1 slice of eggplant vertically on work surface. Place another slice of eggplant crosswise over top to form a cross. Put 1 1/2 tsp. (7 mL) pesto in centre of cross. Sprinkle 3 tbsp. (50 mL) cheese over pesto. Place 2 tbsp. (30 mL) red pepper on top. Fold eggplant ends into centre to enclose filling. Turn over. Place, folded-side down, on greased baking sheet with sides. Repeat with remaining eggplant and fillings.

Brush olive oil over envelopes. Sprinkle with salt and pepper. Bake for about 15 minutes until filling is hot and eggplant starts to turn golden. Serves 4.

*1 serving: 117 Calories; 8.5 g Total Fat (5.0 g Mono, 0.7 g Poly, 2.0 g Sat); 5 mg Cholesterol; 8 g Carbohydrate; 4 g Fibre; 4 g Protein; 188 mg Sodium*

 *fyi*  Fibre, fibre everywhere—but make sure you have lots to drink! To get the full digestive benefits of fibre, you need to accompany it with plenty of fluids. If you eat a lot of fibre but don't drink enough liquids, it will take much longer to move through your body.

# Enchilada Casserole

*Lazy day enchiladas! Layers of whole-wheat tortillas surround sweet potato and black bean filling. Great taste with minimal effort!*

| | | |
|---|---|---|
| Whole-wheat flour tortillas (9 inch, 22 cm, diameter), quartered | 4 | 4 |
| Can of sweet potatoes, drained | 19 oz. | 540 mL |
| Can of black beans, rinsed and drained | 19 oz. | 540 mL |
| Chunky mild salsa | 1/2 cup | 125 mL |
| Chili powder | 2 tsp. | 10 mL |
| Can of tomato sauce | 14 oz. | 398 mL |
| Chunky mild salsa | 1/2 cup | 125 mL |
| Grated light sharp Cheddar cheese | 1 cup | 250 mL |
| Ripe large avocado, diced | 1 | 1 |
| Finely chopped green onion | 1/4 cup | 60 mL |
| Light sour cream | 1/2 cup | 125 mL |

Preheat oven to 450°F (230°C). Arrange half of tortilla pieces in bottom of greased 9 × 13 inch (22 × 33 cm) baking dish.

Mash sweet potatoes in medium bowl. Add next 3 ingredients. Stir. Spread evenly over tortillas in baking dish. Arrange remaining tortilla pieces over top.

Combine tomato sauce and second amount of salsa in small bowl. Pour evenly over tortillas. Bake, uncovered, in oven for 15 minutes. Sprinkle with cheese. Bake for another 5 minutes until heated through and cheese is golden.

Sprinkle avocado and green onion over top.

Serve with sour cream. Serves 6.

*1 serving: 465 Calories; 11.4 g Total Fat (3.4 g Mono, 1.3 g Poly, 4.1 g Sat); 17 mg Cholesterol; 81 g Carbohydrate; 14 g Fibre; 21 g Protein; 1294 mg Sodium*

Pictured on page 72.

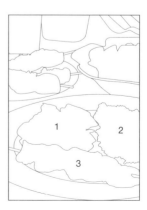

1. Thai Cucumber Salad, page 49
2. Citrus Spice Quinoa Pilaf, page 130
3. Sesame Pork Skewers, page 115

Props courtesy of: Mikasa Home Store
Danesco Inc.

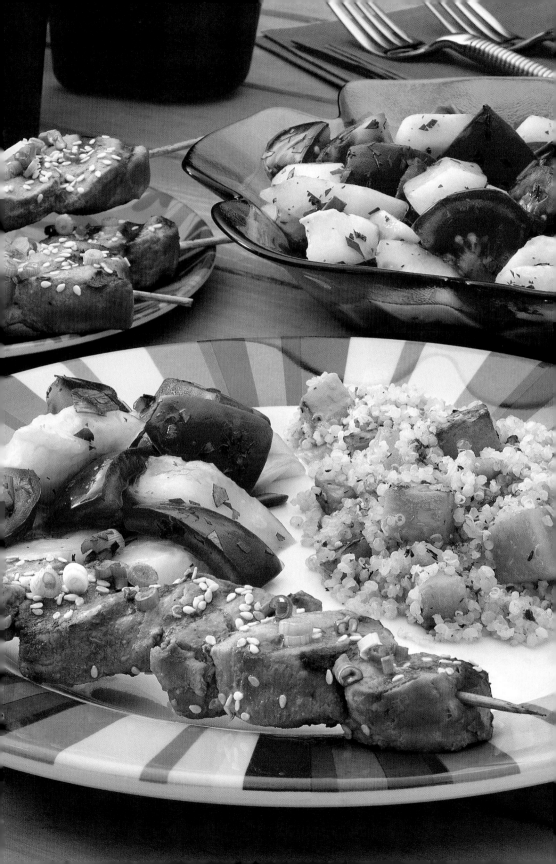

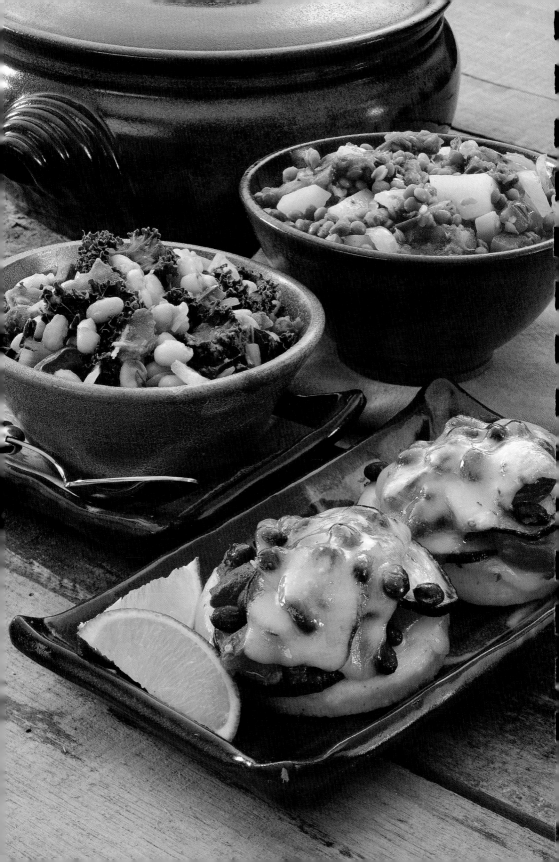

# Polenta Vegetable Stacks

*Plenty of polenta piled high with grilled vegetables and black beans makes for fast, fresh and healthy comfort food. Try adding some Creamy Chipotle Dressing, page 44, for a zippy southwestern flavour. Store your extra polenta, tightly wrapped, in the fridge for up to one month.*

| | | |
|---|---|---|
| Olive oil | 1 tbsp. | 15 mL |
| Tube of plain polenta (2.2 lbs., 1 kg), cut into 8 rounds, about 1/2 inch (12 mm) thick | 1/2 | 1/2 |
| Slices of jalapeño Monterey Jack cheese (about 6 oz., 170 g), cut in half | 8 | 8 |
| Olive oil | 1 tbsp. | 15 mL |
| Thinly sliced zucchini | 1 1/2 cups | 375 mL |
| Garlic cloves, minced (or 1/2 tsp., 2 mL, powder) | 2 | 2 |
| Can of diced tomatoes, drained | 14 oz. | 398 mL |
| Canned black beans, rinsed and drained | 1 cup | 250 mL |

Lime wedges, for garnish

Preheat broiler. Heat first amount of olive oil in large frying pan on medium-high. Add polenta rounds. Cook for about 2 minutes per side until golden. Transfer to greased 9 × 13 inch (22 × 33 cm) baking dish.

Place half slice of cheese on each polenta round. Cover to keep warm.

Heat second amount of olive oil in same frying pan on medium. Add zucchini and garlic. Cook for about 3 minutes until zucchini is tender-crisp.

Add tomatoes and beans. Cook for about 1 minute until heated through. Spoon over polenta. Place remaining cheese slices on top. Broil on centre rack in oven for about 2 minutes until cheese is melted.

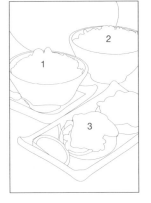

Garnish with lime wedges. Makes 8 stacks. Serves 4.

*1 serving:* 387 Calories; 20.3 g Total Fat (8.7 g Mono, 1.1 g Poly, 9.1 g Sat); 38 mg Cholesterol; 36 g Carbohydrate; 4 g Fibre; 17 g Protein; 562 mg Sodium

Pictured at left.

1. Navy Bean Stew, page 110
2. Cumin Lentils, page 111
3. Polenta Vegetable Stacks, above

Props courtesy of: Out of the Fire Studio

Meatless

# Navy Bean Stew

*You don't have to enlist to enjoy this fresh and hearty stew. Add a slice of lemon for a tiny bit of tang. Serve over soft polenta or with crusty focaccia bread and salad to make this a complete meal.*

| | | |
|---|---|---|
| Canola (or olive) oil | 2 tsp. | 10 mL |
| Chopped onion | 1 1/2 cups | 375 mL |
| Chopped red pepper | 1 1/2 cups | 375 mL |
| Chopped fresh rosemary | 1 tbsp. | 15 mL |
| (or 3/4 tsp., 4 mL, dried, crushed) | | |
| Dried crushed chilies | 1/2 tsp. | 2 mL |
| Garlic cloves, minced | 2 | 2 |
| (or 1/2 tsp., 2 mL, powder) | | |
| Cans of navy beans, rinsed and drained | 2 | 2 |
| (14 oz., 398 mL, each) | | |
| Can of diced tomatoes (with juice) | 14 oz. | 398 mL |
| Water | 1 cup | 250 mL |
| Bay leaf | 1 | 1 |
| Coarsely chopped kale leaves, | 6 cups | 1.5 L |
| lightly packed (see Tip, below) | | |
| Chopped fresh parsley | 1 tbsp. | 15 mL |
| Grated lemon zest | 1 tsp. | 5 mL |

Heat canola oil in large frying pan on medium. Add onion and red pepper. Cook for about 5 minutes, stirring occasionally, until onion starts to soften.

Add next 3 ingredients. Heat and stir for 1 minute until fragrant.

Add next 4 ingredients. Bring to a boil. Reduce heat to medium-low. Simmer, covered, for 10 minutes to blend flavours.

Add kale. Stir. Simmer, covered, for about 3 minutes until kale is wilted. Discard bay leaf.

Add parsley and lemon zest. Stir. Makes about 7 cups (1.75 L).

*1 cup (250 mL): 195 Calories; 2.3 g Total Fat (0.8 g Mono, 0.8 g Poly, 0.3 g Sat); 0 mg Cholesterol; 36 g Carbohydrate; 8 g Fibre; 11 g Protein; 389 mg Sodium*

Pictured on page 108.

  To remove the centre rib from lettuce or kale, fold the leaf in half along the rib and then cut along the length of the rib.

**110**

# Cumin Lentils

*A mild, but far from tame, introduction to curry flavours and meatless eating. This appetizing and colourful blend of lentils, potatoes, tomatoes and spice is excellent served with warm naan bread or whole-wheat pitas.*

| | | |
|---|---|---|
| Diced peeled potato | 2 cups | 500 mL |
| Canola oil | 4 tsp. | 20 mL |
| Thinly sliced onion | 2 cups | 500 mL |
| Thinly sliced celery | 1 cup | 250 mL |
| Ground cumin | 1 tsp. | 5 mL |
| Turmeric | 1/2 tsp. | 2 mL |
| Garlic cloves, minced | 2 | 2 |
|   (or 1/2 tsp., 2 mL, powder) | | |
| Pepper | 1/4 tsp. | 1 mL |
| Cans of lentils, rinsed and drained | 2 | 2 |
|   (19 oz., 540 mL, each) | | |
| Chopped tomato | 2 cups | 500 mL |
|   Prepared vegetable broth | 1 cup | 250 mL |
| Chopped fresh parsley (or cilantro), | | |
|   for garnish | | |

Put potato into microwave-safe dish. Microwave, covered, on high (100%) for about 6 minutes until tender.

Meanwhile, heat canola oil in large frying pan on medium-high. Add onion and celery. Cook for 5 to 10 minutes, stirring often, until onion starts to brown.

Add next 4 ingredients. Heat and stir for 1 minute until fragrant.

Add next 3 ingredients and potato. Stir. Reduce heat to medium. Cook, covered, for about 5 minutes, stirring occasionally, until celery is softened.

Garnish with parsley. Makes about 8 cups (2 L).

*1 cup (250 mL): 220 Calories; 3.0 g Total Fat (1.4 g Mono, 1.0 g Poly, 0.3 g Sat); 0 mg Cholesterol; 39 g Carbohydrate; 7 g Fibre; 12 g Protein; 347 mg Sodium*

Pictured on page 108.

# Cashew Tofu Stir-Fry

*Colourful, crunchy and full of vegetable goodness! Serve over rice for a complete meal.*

| | | |
|---|---|---|
| Water | 3/4 cup | 175 mL |
| Sweet (or regular) chili sauce | 2 tbsp. | 30 mL |
| Cornstarch | 1 tbsp. | 15 mL |
| Soy sauce | 1 tbsp. | 15 mL |
| Sesame oil (optional) | 1 tbsp. | 15 mL |
| Canola oil | 1 tbsp. | 15 mL |
| Chopped suey choy (Chinese cabbage) | 4 cups | 1 L |
| Sugar snap peas, trimmed | 2 cups | 500 mL |
| Sliced onion | 1 1/2 cups | 375 mL |
| Sliced red pepper | 1 cup | 250 mL |
| Finely grated ginger root (or 3/4 tsp., 4 mL, ground ginger) | 1 tbsp. | 15 mL |
| Package of extra-firm tofu, cut into 3/4 inch (2 cm) pieces | 12 1/2 oz. | 350 g |
| Salted cashews | 1/2 cup | 125 mL |

Combine first 5 ingredients in small bowl. Set aside.

Heat large frying pan or wok on medium-high until very hot. Add canola oil. Add next 5 ingredients. Stir-fry for about 2 minutes until vegetables start to soften.

Add tofu and cashews. Stir-fry for 2 to 3 minutes until vegetables are tender-crisp. Stir cornstarch mixture. Add to vegetable mixture. Stir-fry for about 1 minute until boiling and thickened. Serves 4.

*1 serving: 297 Calories; 16.6 g Total Fat (8.3 g Mono, 4.8 g Poly, 2.6 g Sat); 0 mg Cholesterol; 27 g Carbohydrate; 5 g Fibre; 13 g Protein; 750 mg Sodium*

 Tofu, made from soybeans, is rich in protein, high in fibre, low in calories and cholesterol-free. Once you've opened the package of this healthy and satisfying fare, change the water daily and make sure to use it within several days. If you note any trace of a sour odour or taste, your tofu should be given a swift burial—in the garbage can!

# Mediterranean Linguine

*Let your taste buds take a stroll on the Mediterranean. The distinctive flavours of sun-dried tomatoes, balsamic vinegar and feta cheese are showcased in this easy-to-prepare, yet sophisticated-tasting delight.*

| | | |
|---|---|---|
| Whole-wheat linguine | 3/4 lb. | 340 g |
| Sun-dried tomatoes in oil, drained and chopped | 3/4 cup | 175 mL |
| Garlic cloves, minced (or 3/4 tsp., 4 mL, powder) | 3 | 3 |
| Dried crushed chilies | 1/2 tsp. | 2 mL |
| Can of artichoke hearts, drained and quartered | 14 oz. | 398 mL |
| Spinach leaves, lightly packed | 6 cups | 1.5 L |
| Balsamic vinegar | 3 tbsp. | 50 mL |
| Chopped fresh basil | 1/4 cup | 60 mL |
| Pine nuts, toasted (see Tip, page 14) | 1/2 cup | 125 mL |
| Crumbled light feta cheese | 1 cup | 250 mL |

Cook pasta in boiling salted water in large uncovered saucepan or Dutch oven for about 10 minutes, stirring occasionally, until tender but firm. Drain. Return to same pot. Cover to keep warm.

Meanwhile, heat next 3 ingredients in large frying pan on medium for 1 minute. Add artichokes and spinach. Heat and stir for about 2 minutes until spinach is wilted.

Add next 3 ingredients. Reduce heat to low. Heat and stir for 1 minute until vinegar is evaporated. Add to pasta. Toss.

Sprinkle with feta cheese. Serves 4.

*1 serving: 623 Calories; 18.5 g Total Fat (5.8 g Mono, 5.4 g Poly, 4.8 g Sat); 13 mg Cholesterol; 95 g Carbohydrate; 19 g Fibre; 33 g Protein; 680 mg Sodium*

# Apricot Jalapeño Pork

*Sweet, tender pork with a lingering heat. For those who like it even spicier, try including the jalapeño seeds and ribs. Excellent served over rice.*

| | | |
|---|---|---|
| Canola oil | 2 tsp. | 10 mL |
| Pork tenderloin, trimmed of fat, halved lengthwise and cut into 1/4 inch (6 mm) slices | 1 lb. | 454 g |
| Pepper | 1/8 tsp. | 0.5 mL |
| Low-sodium prepared chicken broth | 1/3 cup | 75 mL |
| Dry (or alcohol-free) white wine | 2 tbsp. | 30 mL |
| Apricot jam | 3 tbsp. | 50 mL |
| Jalapeño pepper, finely diced (see Tip, below) | 1 | 1 |

**Chopped fresh cilantro or parsley, for garnish**

Heat canola oil in large frying pan on medium-high. Sprinkle pork with pepper. Add to frying pan. Cook for about 5 minutes, stirring often, until no longer pink inside. Remove to plate. Cover to keep warm.

Add broth and wine to same frying pan. Reduce heat to medium-low. Stir, scraping any brown bits from bottom of pan.

Add jam and jalapeño pepper. Cook and stir for 4 to 5 minutes until sauce is reduced by about half. Spoon over pork.

Garnish with cilantro. Serves 4.

*1 serving: 207 Calories; 5.2 g Total Fat (2.7 g Mono, 1.0 g Poly, 1.2 g Sat); 67 mg Cholesterol; 10 g Carbohydrate; trace Fibre; 27 g Protein; 66 mg Sodium*

Pictured on page 18.

 *tip* Hot peppers contain capsaicin in the seeds and ribs. Removing the seeds and ribs will reduce the heat. Wear rubber gloves when handling hot peppers and avoid touching your eyes. Wash your hands well afterwards.

# Sesame Pork Skewers

*The easiest way to make a weekday meal look special? Skewer it! Tender pork skewers with the classic Asian flavours of ginger, garlic and sesame.*

| | | |
|---|---|---|
| Low-sodium prepared chicken broth | 1/4 cup | 60 mL |
| Sesame oil | 1 tsp. | 5 mL |
| Low-sodium soy sauce | 1 tsp. | 5 mL |
| Rice vinegar | 1 tsp. | 5 mL |
| Brown sugar, packed | 1 tsp. | 5 mL |
| Ground ginger | 1/4 tsp. | 1 mL |
| Garlic powder | 1/4 tsp. | 1 mL |
| Pork tenderloin, trimmed of fat, cut into 3/4 inch (2 cm) cubes | 1 lb. | 454 g |
| Bamboo skewers (8 inches, 20 cm, each), soaked in water for 10 minutes | 4 | 4 |
| Thinly sliced green onion | 2 tbsp. | 30 mL |
| Sesame seeds | 1 1/2 tsp. | 7 mL |

Preheat gas barbecue to medium-high. Combine first 7 ingredients in medium bowl.

Add pork. Toss well. Thread pork onto skewers. Cook on greased grill for about 12 minutes, turning occasionally and basting at halftime with any remaining soy sauce mixture, until no longer pink inside. Remove from heat. Let stand, covered, for 5 minutes.

Sprinkle with green onion and sesame seeds. Makes 4 skewers.

*1 skewer: 166 Calories; 4.5 g Total Fat (1.9 g Mono, 1.0 g Poly, 1.2 g Sat); 67 mg Cholesterol; 2 g Carbohydrate; trace Fibre; 28 g Protein; 101 mg Sodium*

Pictured on page 107.

# Lemon Herb Pork

*Pucker up people, this is a must-try for lemon lovers! Zesty lemon and tarragon sauce coats fork-tender pork medallions.*

| | | |
|---|---|---|
| Olive oil | 1 tbsp. | 15 mL |
| Pork tenderloin, trimmed of fat, cut into 1/4 inch (6 mm) thick slices | 1 lb. | 454 g |
| Slices of lemon, halved crosswise | 4 | 4 |
| Chopped fresh parsley (or 1 1/2 tsp., 7 mL, flakes) | 2 tbsp. | 30 mL |
| Chopped fresh tarragon (or 3/4 tsp., 4 mL, dried) | 1 tbsp. | 15 mL |
| Grated lemon zest | 2 tsp. | 10 mL |
| Garlic clove, minced (or 1/4 tsp., 1 mL, powder) | 1 | 1 |
| Dry (or alcohol-free) white wine | 1/4 cup | 60 mL |
| Evaporated milk | 1/4 cup | 60 mL |
| Salt | 1/2 tsp. | 2 mL |
| Pepper | 1/4 tsp. | 1 mL |

Heat olive oil in large frying pan on medium-high. Add pork. Cook for about 1 minute per side until starting to brown. Remove to plate. Cover to keep warm.

Reduce heat to medium. Add next 5 ingredients to same frying pan. Cook and stir for about 1 minute until garlic is golden.

Add wine. Bring to a boil. Cook for about 1 minute until wine is reduced by half.

Add remaining 3 ingredients and pork. Cook and stir until pork is heated through. Serves 4.

*1 serving: 213 Calories; 7.5 g Total Fat (4.2 g Mono, 0.6 g Poly, 2.2 g Sat); 72 mg Cholesterol; 4 g Carbohydrate; trace Fibre; 28 g Protein; 314 mg Sodium*

# Pork And Sweet Potato Toss

*Take a trip to the islands with this mild introduction to Caribbean flavours!*
*Jerk-seasoned pork and sweet potatoes are tempered by the sweetness of apple.*
*Try the jerk seasoning on chicken too!*

**JERK SEASONING**

| | | |
|---|---|---|
| Onion powder | 1 tsp. | 5 mL |
| Ground thyme | 1/2 tsp. | 2 mL |
| Ground allspice | 1/4 tsp. | 1 mL |
| Pepper | 1/4 tsp. | 1 mL |
| Cayenne pepper | 1/4 tsp. | 1 mL |
| Ground cinnamon | 1/8 tsp. | 0.5 mL |

**PORK AND POTATOES**

| | | |
|---|---|---|
| Canola oil | 1 tbsp. | 15 mL |
| Pork tenderloin, trimmed of fat, halved lengthwise and cut into 1/4 inch (6 mm) slices | 1 lb. | 454 g |
| Chopped peeled sweet potato (or yam) | 3 cups | 750 mL |
| Coleslaw mix | 2 cups | 500 mL |
| Low-sodium prepared chicken broth | 2 tbsp. | 30 mL |
| Medium cooking apples (such as McIntosh), peeled and sliced | 2 | 2 |
| Low-sodium prepared chicken broth | 1/4 cup | 60 mL |
| Golden corn syrup | 2 tbsp. | 30 mL |

**Jerk Seasoning:** Combine all 6 ingredients in small cup. Makes about 2 tsp. (10 mL) seasoning. Set aside.

**Pork And Potatoes:** Heat canola oil in large frying pan or wok on medium-high. Sprinkle pork with 1/4 tsp. (1 mL) Jerk Seasoning. Add to frying pan. Stir-fry for about 5 minutes until no longer pink.

Add next 3 ingredients. Sprinkle with remaining Jerk Seasoning. Reduce heat to medium. Cook, covered, for about 6 minutes, stirring occasionally, until sweet potato starts to soften.

Add remaining 3 ingredients. Stir. Cook, covered, for 2 to 3 minutes, stirring occasionally, until apple is tender. Serves 4.

*1 serving: 315 Calories; 6.6 g Total Fat (3.3 g Mono, 1.5 g Poly, 1.3 g Sat); 67 mg Cholesterol; 35 g Carbohydrate; 4 g Fibre; 30 g Protein; 109 mg Sodium*

# Pear Chutney Pork Chops

*Sugar and spice make these pork chops extra nice! This mild curry is tempered by sweet pear. A perfect dish for those who are new to curry flavours.*

| | | |
|---|---|---|
| All-purpose flour | 1 tbsp. | 15 mL |
| Curry powder | 1 tsp. | 5 mL |
| Ground cardamom | 1/2 tsp. | 2 mL |
| Salt | 1/2 tsp. | 2 mL |
| Pepper | 1/4 tsp. | 1 mL |
| Boneless pork loin chops, trimmed of fat (about 1 lb., 454 g) | 4 | 4 |
| Canola (or olive) oil | 2 tsp. | 10 mL |
| Reserved pear syrup | 1/2 cup | 125 mL |
| Brown sugar, packed | 3 tbsp. | 50 mL |
| Apple cider vinegar | 3 tbsp. | 50 mL |
| Soy sauce | 2 tbsp. | 30 mL |
| Can of pear halves in light syrup, drained and syrup reserved, chopped | 28 oz. | 796 mL |

Combine first 5 ingredients in shallow bowl. Remove half of flour mixture to small bowl. Set aside. Press both sides of pork chops into remaining flour mixture until coated.

Heat canola oil in large frying pan on medium. Add pork chops. Cook for 3 to 4 minutes per side until no longer pink inside. Remove chops to serving plate. Cover to keep warm.

Add next 4 ingredients to reserved flour mixture. Stir with whisk until smooth. Add to frying pan. Heat and stir until boiling and slightly thickened.

Add pears. Stir. Bring to a boil. Reduce heat to medium-low. Simmer, uncovered, for about 5 minutes until slightly thickened. Spoon over chops. Serves 4.

*1 serving: 353 Calories; 8.9 g Total Fat (4.3 g Mono, 1.4 g Poly, 2.4 g Sat); 72 mg Cholesterol; 44 g Carbohydrate; 3 g Fibre; 25 g Protein; 967 mg Sodium*

# Pork Chops Cacciatore

*A delicious and versatile tomato sauce crowns tender pork. The sauce is perfect served over rice or pasta, and makes a quick and healthy alternative to ready-made pasta sauces.*

| | | |
|---|---|---|
| Canola oil | 2 tsp. | 10 mL |
| All-purpose flour | 2 tbsp. | 30 mL |
| Pepper, sprinkle | | |
| Boneless fast-fry pork chops (about 1 lb., 454 g) | 4 | 4 |
| Chopped red pepper | 1 1/2 cups | 375 mL |
| Chopped onion | 1 cup | 250 mL |
| Garlic cloves, minced | 2 | 2 |
| Dry (or alcohol-free) white wine | 1/4 cup | 60 mL |
| Can of diced tomatoes (with juice) | 14 oz. | 398 mL |
| Low-sodium prepared chicken broth | 1/2 cup | 125 mL |
| Brown sugar, packed | 1 tbsp. | 15 mL |
| Dried oregano | 1 tsp. | 5 mL |
| Dried basil | 1/2 tsp. | 2 mL |

Heat canola oil in large frying pan on medium. Meanwhile, combine flour and pepper in small shallow dish. Press both sides of pork into flour mixture until coated. Add to frying pan. Cook for about 4 minutes per side until browned. Remove to plate.

Add next 3 ingredients to same frying pan. Cook for 5 to 10 minutes, stirring often, until onion is softened.

Add wine, scraping any brown bits from bottom of pan.

Add remaining 5 ingredients. Stir. Add pork chops to frying pan. Simmer, uncovered, for about 5 minutes until pork chops are heated through. Serves 4.

*1 serving: 263 Calories; 9.5 g Total Fat (4.4 g Mono, 1.4 g Poly, 2.7 g Sat); 67 mg Cholesterol; 18 g Carbohydrate; 2 g Fibre; 24 g Protein; 317 mg Sodium*

# Five-Spice Pork Medallions

*Five flavours in one spice—you gotta love it! The exotic five-spice crumb coating is wonderful with these tender medallions. Serve with peach-flavoured applesauce for a delicious combination of flavours.*

| | | |
|---|---|---|
| All-purpose flour | 1/3 cup | 75 mL |
| Large egg | 1 | 1 |
| Water | 1 tbsp. | 15 mL |
| Fine dry bread crumbs | 1 cup | 250 mL |
| Chinese five-spice powder | 1 tbsp. | 15 mL |
| Pork tenderloin, trimmed of fat, cut diagonally into 1/4 inch (6 mm) slices | 1 lb. | 454 g |
| Cooking spray | | |
| Salt, sprinkle | | |

Measure flour into shallow bowl. Set aside.

Beat egg and water with fork in small bowl. Set aside.

Preheat oven to 425°F (220°C). Combine bread crumbs and five-spice powder in large resealable freezer bag.

Press each pork slice into flour until lightly coated. Dip into egg mixture. Add, a few at a time, to freezer bag with crumb mixture. Seal bag. Shake until evenly coated. Place on greased baking sheet with sides.

Spray pork with cooking spray. Sprinkle with salt. Bake for 10 to 15 minutes until no longer pink inside. Serves 4.

*1 serving: 309 Calories; 5.9 g Total Fat (2.5 g Mono, 0.8 g Poly, 1.7 g Sat); 113 mg Cholesterol; 29 g Carbohydrate; 1 g Fibre; 33 g Protein; 305 mg Sodium*

 Pork is an excellent source of zinc, which may be one of the most important minerals for food lovers—it helps maintain your senses of smell and taste!

# Peach Basil Pork Chops

*A taste of summer—with a fresh and appetizing presentation.*
*Use fresh peaches when they are in season, and substitute chicken*
*broth for the peach juice.*

| | | |
|---|---|---|
| Canola oil | 1 tbsp. | 15 mL |
| Italian seasoning | 1/2 tsp. | 2 mL |
| Paprika | 1/2 tsp. | 2 mL |
| Salt, sprinkle | | |
| Boneless pork loin chops, trimmed of fat | 4 | 4 |
| (about 1 lb., 454 g) | | |
| Chopped onion | 1/4 cup | 60 mL |
| Apple cider vinegar | 2 tbsp. | 30 mL |
| Can of sliced peaches in juice, drained | 14 oz. | 398 mL |
| and juice reserved | | |
| Reserved peach juice | 1/4 cup | 60 mL |
| Chopped fresh basil | 2 tbsp. | 30 mL |

Heat canola oil in large frying pan on medium-high. Combine next
3 ingredients in small cup. Sprinkle on both sides of pork chops. Add pork
chops to frying pan. Cook for about 2 minutes until browned. Reduce heat
to medium. Turn chops. Cook for about 3 minutes until no longer pink.
Remove to plate. Cover to keep warm.

Add onion to same frying pan. Cook and stir for 1 minute. Add vinegar.
Stir, scraping any brown bits from bottom of pan. Add peaches and
reserved juice. Cook and stir for about 2 minutes until heated through.

Add basil. Stir. Pour over pork chops. Serves 4.

*1 serving: 248 Calories; 11.0 g Total Fat (5.4 g Mono, 1.7 g Poly, 2.9 g Sat); 62 mg Cholesterol;*
*14 g Carbohydrate; 2 g Fibre; 24 g Protein; 49 mg Sodium*

# Roasted Brussels Sprouts

*Just toss together and bake! Roasting brings out the sweetness of vegetables for an easy and delicious side dish.*

| | | |
|---|---|---|
| Frozen baby Brussels sprouts (do not thaw) | 4 cups | 1 L |
| Sliced red onion, cut 1/4 inch (6 mm) thick | 1/2 cup | 125 mL |
| Diced cooked ham | 1/2 cup | 125 mL |
| Olive oil | 1 tbsp. | 15 mL |
| Salt, sprinkle | | |
| Pepper, sprinkle | | |

Preheat oven to 400°F (205°C). Combine all 6 ingredients in large bowl. Toss well. Arrange in single layer on large greased baking sheet with sides. Bake in oven for about 20 minutes, stirring once at halftime, until Brussels sprouts are tender. Serves 6.

*1 serving: 85 Calories; 4.5 g Total Fat (2.6 g Mono, 0.6 g Poly, 1.1 g Sat); 7 mg Cholesterol; 7 g Carbohydrate; 3 g Fibre; 6 g Protein; 146 mg Sodium*

# Honey-Roasted Carrots

*These honey-kissed carrots are a guaranteed hit for those with a sweet tooth.*

| | | |
|---|---|---|
| Baby carrots | 2 lbs. | 900 g |
| Liquid honey | 2 tbsp. | 30 mL |
| Olive oil | 2 tsp. | 10 mL |
| Salt, sprinkle | | |
| Pepper, sprinkle | | |

Preheat oven to 450°F (230°C). Combine all 5 ingredients in large bowl. Toss well. Arrange in single layer on greased baking sheet with sides. Bake in oven for about 15 minutes until tender-crisp. Serves 4.

*1 serving: 140 Calories; 3.5 g Total Fat (1.7 g Mono, 0.8 g Poly, 0.5 g Sat); 0 mg Cholesterol; 27 g Carbohydrate; 4 g Fibre; 2 g Protein; 79 mg Sodium*

# Fragrant Rice

*Subtle Asian-influenced aromas give this dish its scent-ual name. You can use converted whole-grain rice in place of converted white rice for added health benefits. Adjust the cooking time accordingly.*

| | | |
|---|---|---|
| Water | 2 cups | 500 mL |
| Converted white rice | 1 cup | 250 mL |
| Salt | 1/4 tsp. | 1 mL |
| Finely chopped celery | 1/4 cup | 60 mL |
| Sliced green onion | 1/4 cup | 60 mL |
| Low-sodium soy sauce | 2 tbsp. | 30 mL |
| Lime juice | 2 tsp. | 10 mL |
| Liquid honey | 2 tsp. | 10 mL |
| Garlic clove, minced | 1 | 1 |
| (or 1/4 tsp., 1 mL, powder) | | |
| Finely grated ginger root | 1 tsp. | 5 mL |
| (or 1/4 tsp., 1 mL, ground ginger) | | |
| Sesame oil (optional) | 1 tsp. | 5 mL |

Chopped green onion, for garnish

Measure first 3 ingredients into small saucepan. Bring to a boil. Reduce heat to medium-low. Simmer, covered, for about 20 minutes, without stirring, until water is absorbed and rice is tender.

Meanwhile, combine next 8 ingredients in small bowl. Add to rice. Stir well. Cover. Let stand for 5 minutes to blend flavours. Fluff with fork.

Garnish with green onion. Serves 4.

*1 serving: 200 Calories; 1.5 g Total Fat (0.5 g Mono, 0.6 g Poly, 0.3 g Sat); 0 mg Cholesterol; 42 g Carbohydrate; 1 g Fibre; 4 g Protein; 371 mg Sodium*

Pictured on front cover.

## Paré Pointer

*Little Timmy made a spectacle of himself when he was at the optometrist's office.*

# Pepper-Sauced Rotini

*A sure-fire attraction, this easy and elegant rotini will delight one and all.*

| | | |
|---|---|---|
| Whole-wheat rotini | 2 cups | 500 mL |
| Large red pepper, quartered | 1 | 1 |
| Garlic clove, peeled | 1 | 1 |
| Lime juice | 2 tbsp. | 30 mL |
| Olive oil | 1 tbsp. | 15 mL |
| Tomato paste (see Tip, page 83) | 2 tsp. | 10 mL |
| Pepper | 1/8 tsp. | 0.5 mL |
| Grated Parmesan cheese | 1/4 cup | 60 mL |

Cook pasta in boiling salted water in large uncovered saucepan for about 10 minutes, stirring occasionally, until tender but firm. Drain, reserving 2 tbsp. (30 mL) cooking water. Return to same pot. Cover to keep warm.

Meanwhile, put red pepper and garlic into small microwave-safe bowl. Microwave, covered, on high (100%) for about 5 minutes until softened. Let stand for 5 minutes. Remove and discard skin from red pepper. Transfer to blender or food processor.

Add next 4 ingredients. Process until smooth.

Add Parmesan cheese, red pepper mixture and reserved cooking water to pasta. Stir well. Serves 4.

*1 serving: 223 Calories; 6.5 g Total Fat (3.1 g Mono, 0.4 g Poly, 1.7 g Sat); 5 mg Cholesterol; 34 g Carbohydrate; 5 g Fibre; 8 g Protein; 129 mg Sodium*

1. Portobellos And Greens, page 40
2. Basil Pesto Pasta, page 134
3. Grilled Pepper Chicken, page 86

Props courtesy of:  Out of the Fire Studio
Pier 1 Imports
The Bay

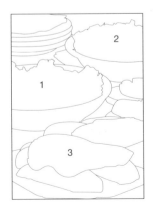

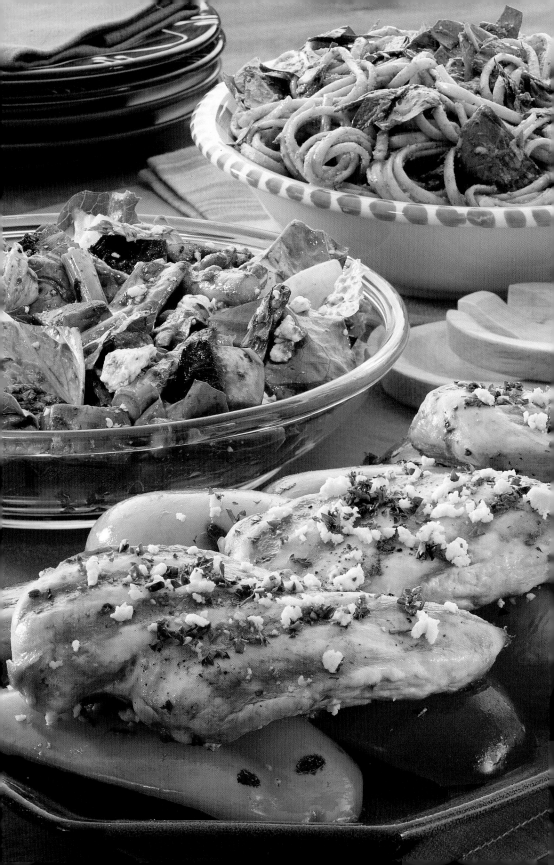

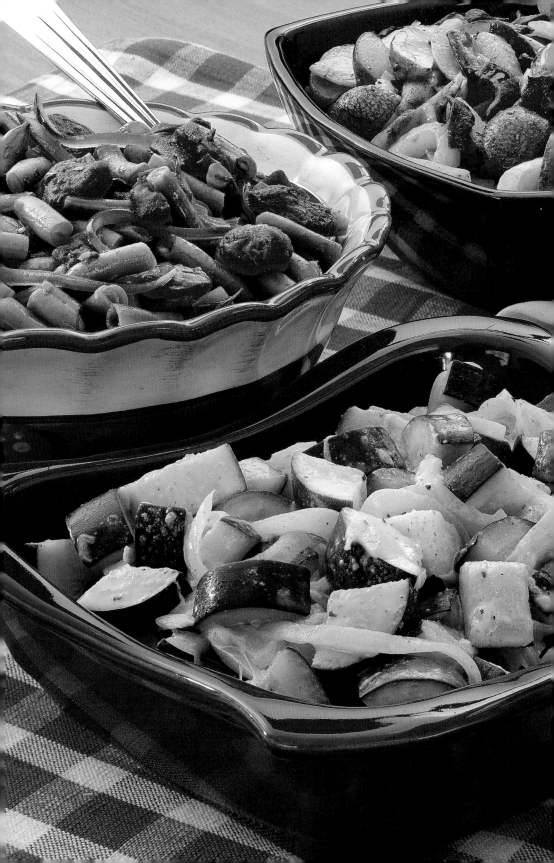

# Rice And Peas Parmesan

*Talk about well-rounded! This side dish covers all your food groups— and has the taste of fresh peas. Use converted whole-grain rice for an added nutty flavour but allow a little longer for cooking.*

| Olive (or canola) oil | 1 tsp. | 5 mL |
|---|---|---|
| Finely chopped onion | 1 cup | 250 mL |
| | | |
| Low-sodium prepared chicken broth | 2 1/4 cups | 550 mL |
| Converted white rice | 1 cup | 250 mL |
| Chopped deli smoked turkey (or ham) slices | 1/2 cup | 125 mL |
| Pepper | 1/4 tsp. | 1 mL |
| | | |
| Frozen peas, thawed (see Tip, page 67) | 1 cup | 250 mL |
| Grated Parmesan cheese | 1/3 cup | 75 mL |
| Chopped fresh parsley | 1/3 cup | 75 mL |

Heat olive oil in medium saucepan on medium-high. Add onion. Cook for about 3 minutes until starting to brown.

Add next 4 ingredients. Bring to a boil. Reduce heat to medium-low. Simmer, covered, for about 20 minutes, without stirring, until rice is tender.

Stir remaining 3 ingredients into rice mixture. Serves 4.

*1 serving: 290 Calories; 4.8 g Total Fat (1.8 g Mono, 0.4 g Poly, 1.9 g Sat); 13 mg Cholesterol; 48 g Carbohydrate; 3 g Fibre; 13 g Protein; 382 mg Sodium*

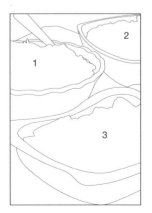

1. Balsamic Beans, page 129
2. Fennel Potatoes, page 128
3. Creamy Curried Zucchini, page 132

Props courtesy of: Cherison Enterprises Inc.
Canhome Global

Sides

# Fennel Potatoes

*Tender vegetables and potatoes tossed together with a hint of lemon pepper and the delicate licorice taste of fennel.*

| | | |
|---|---|---|
| Olive oil | 2 tbsp. | 30 mL |
| Thinly sliced fennel bulb (white part only) | 2 cups | 500 mL |
| Red baby potatoes, cut into 8 wedges each | 1 lb. | 454 g |
| Lemon pepper | 1/2 tsp. | 2 mL |
| Roasted red pepper, drained and blotted dry, cut into strips | 1 cup | 250 mL |
| Prepared chicken broth | 3 tbsp. | 50 mL |

Heat olive oil in large frying pan on medium-high. Add next 3 ingredients. Cook for about 5 minutes, stirring often, until potato and fennel start to brown.

Add red pepper and broth. Stir. Reduce heat to medium. Cook, covered, for about 10 minutes, stirring occasionally, until potato is tender. Serves 4.

*1 serving: 213 Calories; 7.4 g Total Fat (5.0 g Mono, 0.7 g Poly, 0.9 g Sat); 0 mg Cholesterol; 35 g Carbohydrate; 8 g Fibre; 5 g Protein; 261 mg Sodium*

Pictured on page 126.

# Tangy Asparagus

*With its white wine, lemon and garlic flavours, this side dish is guaranteed to impress even the most refined of guests!*

| | | |
|---|---|---|
| Olive oil | 2 tbsp. | 30 mL |
| Finely chopped onion | 1/2 cup | 125 mL |
| Garlic cloves, minced (or 1/2 tsp., 2 mL, powder) | 2 | 2 |
| Fresh asparagus, trimmed of tough ends and cut into 2 inch (5 cm) pieces | 2 lbs. | 900 g |
| Dry (or alcohol-free) white wine | 1/4 cup | 60 mL |
| Lemon juice | 1/4 cup | 60 mL |
| Salt, sprinkle | | |
| Pepper, sprinkle | | |

*(continued on next page)*

Heat olive oil in large frying pan on medium. Add onion and garlic. Cook for about 2 minutes until onion starts to soften.

Add asparagus. Cook and stir for about 3 minutes until almost tender-crisp.

Add remaining 4 ingredients. Heat and stir for 1 minute to blend flavours. Serves 4.

*1 serving: 139 Calories; 7.2 g Total Fat (5.0 g Mono, 0.8 g Poly, 1.0 g Sat); 0 mg Cholesterol; 15 g Carbohydrate; 4 g Fibre; 6 g Protein; 6 mg Sodium*

# Balsamic Beans

*Complementary colours of red and green make this dish appealing to the eye. Complementary flavours of beans and balsamic vinegar make this dish appealing to the palate.*

| | | |
|---|---|---|
| Frozen cut green beans | 5 cups | 1.25 L |
| Olive oil | 1 tbsp. | 15 mL |
| Thinly sliced red onion | 1/4 cup | 60 mL |
| Garlic clove, minced | 1 | 1 |
| (or 1/4 tsp., 1 mL, powder) | | |
| Can of diced tomatoes, drained | 14 oz. | 398 mL |
| Balsamic vinegar | 3 tbsp. | 50 mL |
| Parsley flakes | 1 tsp. | 5 mL |
| Dried basil | 1/2 tsp. | 2 mL |

Cook beans in boiling salted water in large partially covered saucepan for about 6 minutes, stirring occasionally, until tender but firm. Drain. Return to same pot. Cover to keep warm.

Meanwhile, heat olive oil in medium frying pan on medium. Add onion and garlic. Cook for about 5 minutes until onion is softened.

Add remaining 4 ingredients. Heat and stir for 2 minutes to blend flavours. Add to beans. Toss. Serves 4.

*1 serving: 108 Calories; 3.5 g Total Fat (2.5 g Mono, 0.3 g Poly, 0.5 g Sat); 0 mg Cholesterol; 16 g Carbohydrate; 5 g Fibre; 3 g Protein; 430 mg Sodium*

Pictured on page 126.

# Citrus Spice Quinoa Pilaf

*You'll be keen on this fluffy quinoa (pronounced KEEN–wah) pilaf scented with lemon and thyme. Quinoa is available in the bulk or health food sections of grocery stores.*

| | | |
|---|---|---|
| Low-sodium prepared chicken broth | 2 cups | 500 mL |
| Quinoa, rinsed and drained | 1 cup | 250 mL |
| Bay leaf | 1 | 1 |
| Olive oil | 1 tbsp. | 15 mL |
| Diced butternut squash | 2 cups | 500 mL |
| Chopped onion | 1 cup | 250 mL |
| Chopped fresh thyme | 2 tsp. | 10 mL |
| (or 1/2 tsp., 2 mL, dried) | | |
| Dried crushed chilies | 1/4 tsp. | 1 mL |
| Salt, sprinkle | | |
| Lemon juice | 2 tbsp. | 30 mL |
| Grated lemon zest (see Tip, page 140) | 2 tsp. | 10 mL |

Combine first 3 ingredients in medium saucepan. Bring to a boil. Reduce heat to medium-low. Simmer, covered, for about 15 minutes until broth is absorbed. Discard bay leaf.

Meanwhile, heat olive oil in large frying pan on medium. Add next 5 ingredients. Cook, covered, for 5 to 10 minutes, stirring occasionally, until squash and onion are softened and lightly browned. Remove from heat.

Add lemon juice, lemon zest and quinoa. Stir. Serves 4.

*1 serving: 272 Calories; 6.4 g Total Fat (3.3 g Mono, 1.4 g Poly, 0.9 g Sat); 0 mg Cholesterol; 49 g Carbohydrate; 6 g Fibre; 8 g Protein; 33 mg Sodium*

Pictured on page 107.

### Paré Pointer

*He's like a skunk. When he gets mad, he raises a stink.*

# Lemon Leek Linguine

*A very intriguing dinner companion (for salmon or chicken, at least) and a very tasty pasta dish for you! Serve immediately.*

| | | |
|---|---|---|
| Whole-wheat linguine | 3/4 lb. | 340 g |
| Olive oil | 2 tsp. | 10 mL |
| Sliced leek (white part only) | 2 cups | 500 mL |
| Garlic cloves, minced | 2 | 2 |
| Low-sodium prepared chicken broth | 1/2 cup | 125 mL |
| Dry (or alcohol-free) white wine | 1/3 cup | 75 mL |
| Grated lemon zest | 2 tsp. | 10 mL |
| Pepper | 1/2 tsp. | 2 mL |
| Evaporated milk | 1/2 cup | 125 mL |
| Grated Parmesan cheese | 1/4 cup | 60 mL |
| Chopped fresh dill | 2 tbsp. | 30 mL |

Cook pasta in boiling salted water in uncovered Dutch oven or large pot for 10 to 12 minutes, stirring occasionally, until tender but firm. Drain, reserving 1/4 cup (60 mL) cooking water. Return to same pot. Cover to keep warm.

Meanwhile, heat olive oil in large frying pan on medium. Add leek and garlic. Cook, covered, for about 5 minutes, stirring occasionally, until leek is softened.

Add next 4 ingredients. Bring to a boil. Heat and stir for 2 minutes.

Add evaporated milk. Stir. Heat until hot, but not boiling. Add to pasta. Add reserved cooking water. Stir well. Transfer to serving bowl.

Sprinkle with Parmesan cheese and dill. Serves 4.

*1 serving:* 423 Calories; 5.7 g Total Fat (2.4 g Mono, 0.8 g Poly, 1.8 g Sat); 5 mg Cholesterol; 78 g Carbohydrate; 9 g Fibre; 17 g Protein; 146 mg Sodium

# Creamy Curried Zucchini

*This is the dish you'll want to invite to all your dinners—it goes well with everything!*

| | | |
|---|---|---|
| Canola oil | 1 tbsp. | 15 mL |
| Thinly sliced onion | 1 cup | 250 mL |
| Curry powder | 1 1/2 tsp. | 7 mL |
| Low-sodium prepared chicken (or vegetable) broth | 1/2 cup | 125 mL |
| Medium zucchini, quartered lengthwise and cut into 1/2 inch (12 mm) pieces | 2 | 2 |
| Salt, sprinkle | | |
| Pepper, sprinkle | | |
| Light spreadable cream cheese | 2 tbsp. | 30 mL |

Heat canola oil in large frying pan on medium-high until very hot. Add onion. Stir-fry for about 2 minutes until starting to turn golden.

Add curry powder. Stir-fry for about 1 minute until fragrant.

Add next 4 ingredients. Stir-fry for about 5 minutes until zucchini is tender-crisp. Remove from heat.

Add cream cheese. Stir well. Serves 4.

*1 serving: 89 Calories; 5.1 g Total Fat (2.1 g Mono, 1.2 g Poly, 1.2 g Sat); 4 mg Cholesterol; 9 g Carbohydrate; 2 g Fibre; 3 g Protein; 56 mg Sodium*

Pictured on page 126.

**Variation:** Use 4 cups (1 L) broccoli or cauliflower florets instead of zucchini.

# Asparagus Spaghetti

*Get a double dose of nutrients with a helping of whole-wheat spaghetti and healthful asparagus. This side dish should please all tastes—it's a little bit sweet and a little bit spicy.*

| | | |
|---|---|---|
| Whole-wheat spaghetti | 8 oz. | 225 g |
| Fresh asparagus, trimmed of tough ends and cut into 2 inch (5 cm) pieces | 1 lb. | 454 g |
| Orange juice | 1 tbsp. | 15 mL |
| Cornstarch | 1 tsp. | 5 mL |
| Olive oil | 2 tsp. | 10 mL |
| Garlic cloves, minced (or 1/2 tsp., 2 mL powder) | 2 | 2 |
| Orange juice | 1 cup | 250 mL |
| Rice vinegar | 2 tsp. | 10 mL |
| Grated lemon zest | 1 tsp. | 5 mL |
| Dried crushed chilies | 1/8 – 1/4 tsp. | 0.5 – 1 mL |

Chopped fresh chives, for garnish

Cook spaghetti in boiling salted water in large uncovered saucepan or Dutch oven for 8 minutes, stirring occasionally. Add asparagus. Stir. Cook for about 3 minutes until spaghetti is tender but firm. Drain. Return to same pot. Cover to keep warm.

Meanwhile, stir first amount of orange juice into cornstarch in small cup. Set aside.

Heat olive oil in small frying pan on medium. Add garlic. Cook for about 2 minutes, stirring occasionally, until fragrant.

Add next 4 ingredients. Stir. Simmer for 5 minutes to blend flavours. Stir cornstarch mixture. Add to garlic mixture. Heat and stir for 1 to 2 minutes until boiling and thickened. Pour over spaghetti and asparagus. Toss well.

Garnish with chives. Serves 6.

*1 serving: 101 Calories; 2.0 g Total Fat (1.2 g Mono, 0.3 g Poly, 0.3 g Sat); 0 mg Cholesterol; 19 g Carbohydrate; 2 g Fibre; 4 g Protein; 3 mg Sodium*

# Basil Pesto Pasta

*Make this in the summer when you harvest your herb garden. A healthier version with less oil than traditional pesto. Excellent with grilled chicken.*

| | | |
|---|---|---|
| Whole-wheat linguine | 8 oz. | 225 g |
| Fresh basil, lightly packed | 1 cup | 250 mL |
| Salted, roasted shelled pumpkin seeds | 1/4 cup | 60 mL |
| Water | 1/4 cup | 60 mL |
| Olive oil | 2 tbsp. | 30 mL |
| Lemon juice | 2 tbsp. | 30 mL |
| Garlic cloves, minced | 2 | 2 |
| (or 1/2 tsp., 2 mL, powder) | | |
| Chopped fresh spinach leaves, lightly packed | 2 cups | 500 mL |
| Grated Parmesan cheese | 1/4 cup | 60 mL |

Cook pasta in boiling salted water in large uncovered saucepan or Dutch oven for about 12 minutes, stirring occasionally, until tender but firm. Drain, reserving 1/2 cup (125 mL) cooking water. Return to same pot. Cover to keep warm.

Meanwhile, process next 6 ingredients in blender or food processor until smooth.

Add spinach, Parmesan cheese and basil mixture to pasta. Toss, adding reserved cooking water a little at a time, if needed, to moisten. Serve immediately. Serves 4.

*1 serving: 372 Calories; 15.6 g Total Fat (7.5 g Mono, 3.8 g Poly, 3.4 g Sat); 5 mg Cholesterol; 47 g Carbohydrate; 6 g Fibre; 17 g Protein; 218 mg Sodium*

Pictured on page 125.

# Butternut Squash Toss

*This toss will never leave you at a loss for what to make for dinner! Its pretty colours and contrasting textures are sure to please the palate.*

| | | |
|---|---|---|
| Butternut squash, cut into 1/2 inch (12 mm) pieces (about 3 cups, 750 mL) | 1 1/2 lbs. | 680 g |
| Balsamic vinegar | 1 tbsp. | 15 mL |
| Brown sugar, packed | 1 tbsp. | 15 mL |
| Olive oil | 2 tsp. | 10 mL |
| Pepper | 1/4 tsp. | 1 mL |
| Fresh spinach leaves, lightly packed, chopped | 3 cups | 750 mL |
| Olive oil | 1 tbsp. | 15 mL |
| Lemon juice | 1 tbsp. | 15 mL |
| Salt, sprinkle | | |
| Raw pumpkin seeds, toasted (see Tip, page 14) | 2 tbsp. | 30 mL |
| Crumbled blue cheese | 1 oz. | 28 g |

Toss first 5 ingredients in large microwave-safe bowl. Microwave, covered, on high (100%) for 10 minutes. Stir. Microwave, covered, for another 3 to 5 minutes until squash is tender-crisp.

Add next 4 ingredients. Stir. Microwave, covered, on high (100%) for 30 seconds until spinach is wilted. Transfer to serving dish.

Sprinkle pumpkin seeds and blue cheese over centre of squash mixture. Serves 4.

*1 serving:* 214 Calories; 10.9 g Total Fat (5.6 g Mono, 2.0 g Poly, 2.7 g Sat); 5 mg Cholesterol; 27 g Carbohydrate; 5 g Fibre; 6 g Protein; 127 mg Sodium

# Tropical Peppers

*This combination of fruit and vegetables makes a colourful side dish that goes well with fish, pork or poultry. Enjoy the simple and mildly sweet flavours of glazed pineapple and bell peppers.*

| | | |
|---|---|---|
| Can of pineapple chunks, drained and juice reserved | 14 oz. | 398 mL |
| Large green pepper, cut into 1 inch (2.5 cm) strips | 1 | 1 |
| Large red pepper, cut into 1 inch (2.5 cm) strips | 1 | 1 |
| Large orange pepper, cut into 1 inch (2.5 cm) strips | 1 | 1 |
| Olive oil | 2 tsp. | 10 mL |
| Salt, sprinkle | | |
| Pepper, sprinkle | | |
| Reserved pineapple juice | 2/3 cup | 150 mL |
| Cornstarch | 1 tsp. | 5 mL |

Preheat broiler. Put first 4 ingredients into large bowl. Drizzle with olive oil. Sprinkle with salt and pepper. Toss well. Arrange pineapple with peppers, skin side up, in single layer on greased baking sheet with sides. Broil on top rack in oven for about 10 minutes until peppers are just starting to blacken and pineapple is hot.

Meanwhile, stir reserved pineapple juice into cornstarch in medium saucepan until smooth. Bring to a boil on medium, stirring constantly, until boiling and thickened. Add peppers and pineapple. Stir until coated. Serves 6.

*1 serving: 89 Calories; 1.8 g Total Fat (1.1 g Mono, 0.2 g Poly, 0.3 g Sat); 0 mg Cholesterol; 19 g Carbohydrate; 2 g Fibre; 1 g Protein; 3 mg Sodium*

Pictured on front cover.

# Black Bean And Corn Skillet

*A great side dish for your next barbecue! This light and colourful dish is very versatile—it can be served at room temperature or chilled. If you like the tangy taste of balsamic or want to really feel the heat in your cayenne, opt for the larger measurement options.*

| | | |
|---|---|---|
| Olive oil | 1 tbsp. | 15 mL |
| Frozen kernel corn | 2 cups | 500 mL |
| Diced zucchini | 3/4 cup | 175 mL |
| Diced red pepper | 1/2 cup | 125 mL |
| Garlic clove, minced | 1 | 1 |
| (or 1/4 tsp., 1 mL, powder) | | |
| Cayenne pepper | 1/8 – 1/4 tsp. | 0.5 – 1 mL |
| Can of black beans, rinsed and drained | 19 oz. | 540 mL |
| Finely chopped green onion | 1/4 cup | 60 mL |
| Balsamic vinegar | 1 – 2 tbsp. | 15 – 30 mL |
| Grated lemon zest | 2 tsp. | 10 mL |
| Chopped fresh thyme | 1 tsp. | 5 mL |
| (or 1/4 tsp., 1 mL, dried) | | |

Heat olive oil in large frying pan on medium. Add next 5 ingredients. Cook for 8 to 10 minutes, stirring occasionally, until vegetables are tender-crisp.

Add remaining 5 ingredients. Heat and stir for 2 minutes to blend flavours. Serves 4.

*1 serving: 299 Calories; 4.8 g Total Fat (2.7 g Mono, 0.9 g Poly, 0.8 g Sat); 0 mg Cholesterol; 53 g Carbohydrate; 12 g Fibre; 15 g Protein; 330 mg Sodium*

Pictured on page 18.

---

## Paré Pointer

*The banana went to see the prune because he couldn't get a date.*

# Quick Fruit Compote

*Very versatile! Serve hot or cold, as a dessert or as a condiment. Makes a great topping for pancakes or yogurt. Doubles easily and keeps well in the refrigerator, so make a big batch to keep on hand for a quick snack.*

| | | |
|---|---|---|
| White grape juice (see Note) | 3/4 cup | 175 mL |
| Coarsely chopped dried apricot | 1/2 cup | 125 mL |
| Large pear, peeled and cut into 1/2 inch (12 mm) pieces | 1 | 1 |
| Medium cooking apple (such as McIntosh), peeled and diced | 1 | 1 |
| Medium orange, peeled and cut into 1/2 inch (12 mm) pieces | 1 | 1 |
| Fresh (or frozen) cranberries | 1 cup | 250 mL |
| Orange liqueur (or orange juice) | 1 tbsp. | 15 mL |

Combine first 4 ingredients in medium saucepan. Bring to a boil. Reduce heat to medium-low. Simmer, uncovered, for about 5 minutes until softened.

Add orange and cranberries. Stir gently. Cook for about 5 minutes until cranberries begin to split.

Stir in liqueur. Makes about 3 cups (750 mL).

*1 cup (250 mL): 204 Calories; 0.3 g Total Fat (trace Mono, 0.1 g Poly, 0.1 g Sat); 0 mg Cholesterol; 50 g Carbohydrate; 7 g Fibre; 2 g Protein; 21 mg Sodium*

**Note:** If necessary, add up to another 1/4 cup (60 mL) white grape juice to get the desired consistency.

**HOLIDAY FRUIT COMPOTE:** Add 2 tbsp. (30 mL) finely chopped crystallized ginger, a 4 inch (10 cm) stick of cinnamon and 4 whole cloves with first 4 ingredients. Discard cinnamon stick and cloves before serving.

 Cranberry may just be your bladder's best friend. It makes your bladder slippery so anything nasty that wants to stick around, attach to your bladder walls and cause problems has a heck of a time hanging on.

# Bread Puddings

*With sweet apples and a kiss of cinnamon, this one's a real beauty. Best served with a scoop of vanilla frozen yogurt.*

| | | |
|---|---|---|
| Chopped dried apple | 1/2 cup | 125 mL |
| Apple juice | 1/4 cup | 60 mL |
| Large eggs | 2 | 2 |
| Can of skim evaporated milk | 13 1/2 oz. | 385 mL |
| Brown sugar, packed | 3 tbsp. | 50 mL |
| Vanilla extract | 1 tsp. | 5 mL |
| Ground cinnamon | 1/2 tsp. | 2 mL |
| Ground nutmeg, sprinkle | | |
| Salt, just a pinch | | |
| Whole-grain bread slices, cubed | 4 | 4 |
| (about 3 cups, 750 mL) | | |
| Brown sugar, packed | 4 tsp. | 20 mL |

Preheat oven to 375°F (190°C). Combine apples and apple juice in small microwave-safe bowl. Microwave, uncovered, on medium (50%) for 45 seconds.

Meanwhile, beat eggs in medium bowl. Stir in next 6 ingredients. Add bread cubes and apple mixture. Stir. Spoon into 4 greased 1 cup (250 mL) ramekins or ovenproof bowls.

Sprinkle with second amount of brown sugar. Place ramekins on baking sheet with sides. Bake in oven for about 20 minutes until top is golden and a knife inserted in centre comes out clean. Let stand for 3 to 4 minutes until set. Serves 4.

*1 serving: 327 Calories; 3.5 g Total Fat (1.5 g Mono, 0.6 g Poly, 1.0 g Sat); 93 mg Cholesterol; 61 g Carbohydrate; 3 g Fibre; 13 g Protein; 433 mg Sodium*

# Dessert Quesadillas

*Guiltless but oh, so good! You can't go wrong with this banana and chocolate-filled whole-wheat quesadilla. Use dark chocolate chips for a healthier choice. Serve with vanilla frozen yogurt. Peanut butter lovers must try the Banana Nut variation!*

| | | |
|---|---|---|
| Granulated sugar | 2 tsp. | 10 mL |
| Ground cinnamon | 1/8 tsp. | 0.5 mL |
| Small bananas, thinly sliced | 2 | 2 |
| Lemon juice | 2 tsp. | 10 mL |
| Whole-wheat flour tortillas (9 inch, 22 cm, diameter) | 4 | 4 |
| Dark (or semi-sweet) chocolate chips | 1/4 cup | 60 mL |

Cooking spray

Preheat oven to 350°F (175°C). Combine sugar and cinnamon in small cup. Set aside.

Put banana slices and lemon juice into small bowl. Toss gently.

Arrange banana slices on half of each tortilla. Sprinkle chocolate chips over banana. Fold tortillas in half to cover filling. Transfer to ungreased baking sheet with sides.

Spray tortillas with cooking spray. Sprinkle cinnamon mixture over top. Bake in oven for about 5 minutes until chocolate chips are melted. Cut tortillas into wedges. Serves 4.

*1 serving: 262 Calories; 6.0 g Total Fat (0.1 g Mono, 0.4 g Poly, 3.2 g Sat); 0 mg Cholesterol; 58 g Carbohydrate; 5 g Fibre; 7 g Protein; 299 mg Sodium*

**BANANA NUT QUESADILLAS:** Spread 1 tbsp. (15 mL) peanut butter on half of each tortilla before arranging banana slices.

 When a recipe calls for both the zest and juice of a citrus fruit, be sure to grate the zest before juicing.

# Orange Soufflé Clouds

*These individual soufflés will have you floating high. Ensure your beaters and bowl are grease-free.*

| | | |
|---|---|---|
| Granulated sugar | 2 tbsp. | 30 mL |
| Skim milk | 1 cup | 250 mL |
| Granulated sugar | 3 tbsp. | 50 mL |
| Cornstarch | 2 tbsp. | 30 mL |
| Egg yolk (large), fork-beaten | 1 | 1 |
| Orange juice | 1/3 cup | 75 mL |
| Grated orange zest (see Tip, page 140) | 1 tbsp. | 15 mL |
| Egg whites (large), room temperature | 5 | 5 |
| Cream of tartar | 1/2 tsp. | 2 mL |
| Granulated sugar | 3 tbsp. | 50 mL |

Preheat oven to 400°F (205°C). Sprinkle first amount of sugar into greased 6 oz. (170 mL) ramekin. Tilt ramekin to coat bottom and sides with sugar. Gently tap excess sugar into another greased ramekin. Repeat 5 more times to prepare a total of 6 sugar-coated ramekins. Discard excess sugar from last ramekin once coated. Place ramekins on baking sheet with sides. Set aside.

Combine next 3 ingredients in small saucepan on medium. Heat and stir for about 5 minutes until boiling and thickened.

Combine next 3 ingredients in small cup. Add to milk mixture, stirring constantly with whisk for about 1 minute until thick. Transfer to medium bowl.

Beat egg whites and cream of tartar in large bowl until soft peaks form. Add third amount of sugar 1 tbsp. (15 mL) at a time, beating constantly until stiff peaks form and sugar is dissolved. Fold about 1/3 of egg white mixture into hot milk mixture until almost combined. Fold milk mixture into remaining egg whites until no white streaks remain. Spoon into ramekins. Smooth tops. Bake in oven for about 12 minutes, without opening oven door, until very puffed and tops are golden. Serves 6.

*1 serving: 117 Calories; 0.9 g Total Fat (0.4 g Mono, 0.1 g Poly, 0.3 g Sat); 32 mg Cholesterol; 22 g Carbohydrate; trace Fibre; 5 g Protein; 68 mg Sodium*

Pictured on page 143.

**TART LEMON SOUFFLÉ CLOUDS:** Use same amounts of lemon juice and lemon zest instead of orange juice and orange zest.

# Melon Banana Splits

*No one's going to split when this fun and fruity treat is served. Think of it as an artistic way of getting your fruit. Refreshing, delicious and very healthy!*

| | | |
|---|---|---|
| **Large bananas, halved crosswise** | 2 | 2 |
| **Chopped watermelon** | 1 1/3 cups | 325 mL |
| **Chopped honeydew** | 1 1/3 cups | 325 mL |
| **Chopped cantaloupe** | 1 1/3 cups | 325 mL |
| **Vanilla yogurt** | 1 cup | 250 mL |
| **Fresh blueberries** | 1/4 cup | 60 mL |
| **Chopped fresh pineapple** (or canned tidbits, drained) | 1/4 cup | 60 mL |
| **Fresh raspberries** | 1/4 cup | 60 mL |
| **Caramel ice cream topping (optional)** | 2 tbsp. | 30 mL |

Cut banana halves lengthwise to make 8 pieces. Place 2 banana pieces on opposite sides of 4 banana split dishes or shallow bowls.

Drop spoonfuls of next 3 ingredients in separate mounds between banana pieces.

Drizzle yogurt over melon.

Sprinkle next 3 ingredients over yogurt.

Drizzle with ice cream topping. Serves 4.

*1 serving: 175 Calories; 1.4 g Total Fat (0.1 g Mono, 0.2 g Poly, 0.6 g Sat); 3 mg Cholesterol; 40 g Carbohydrate; 3 g Fibre; 4 g Protein; 54 mg Sodium*

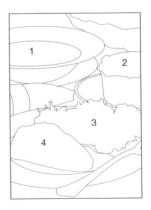

1. Sweet Pea Soup, page 58
2. Orange Soufflé Clouds, page 141
3. Summer Salad, page 43
4. Tarragon-Poached Fish, page 91

Props courtesy of: Mikasa Home Store
Dansk Gifts
Pfaltzgraff Canada

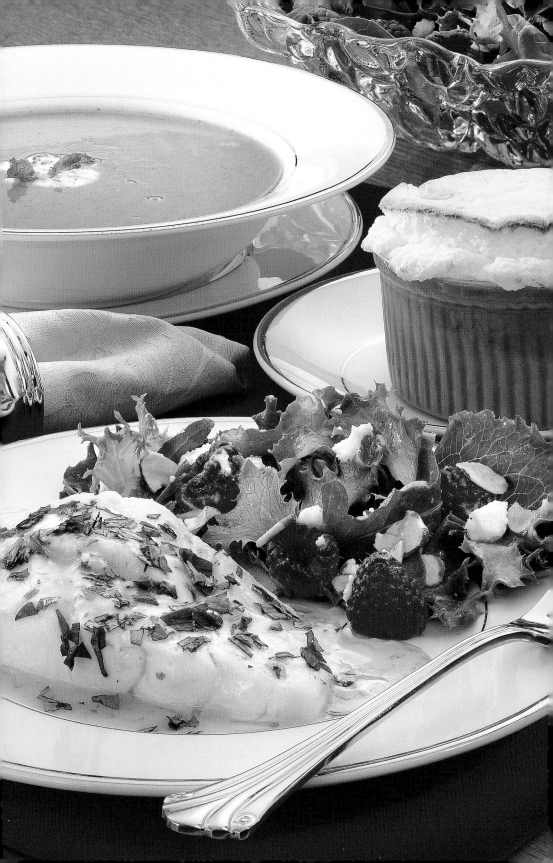

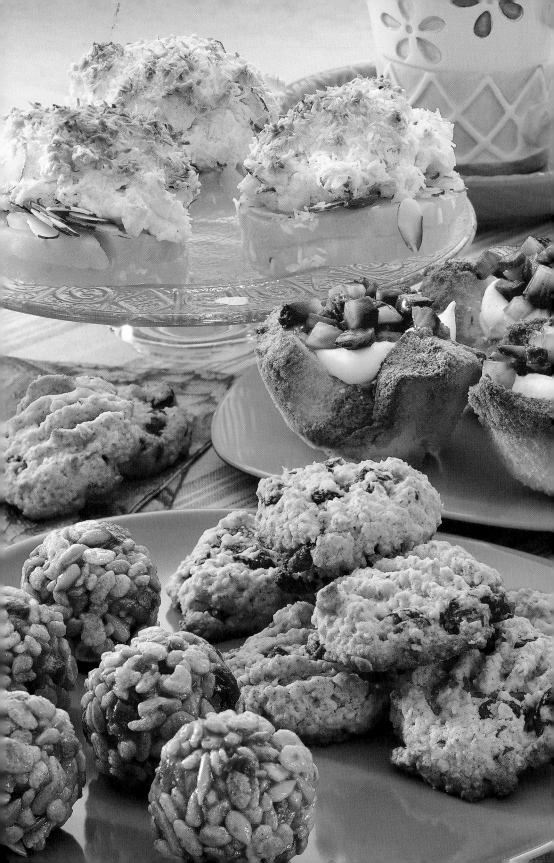

# Oatmeal Cranberry Cookies

*Quell the inner cookie monster when a craving hits. Full of oats, wheat germ, pecans and cranberries, this cookie is a guilt-free treat. A small ice cream scoop helps portion the dough quickly and evenly.*

| | | |
|---|---|---|
| Butter (or hard margarine), softened | 1/2 cup | 125 mL |
| Brown sugar, packed | 1/2 cup | 125 mL |
| Large egg | 1 | 1 |
| Vanilla extract | 1/2 tsp. | 2 mL |
| Quick-cooking rolled oats | 1 cup | 250 mL |
| All-purpose flour | 2/3 cup | 150 mL |
| Wheat germ | 1/2 cup | 125 mL |
| Baking powder | 1 tsp. | 5 mL |
| Salt | 1/2 tsp. | 2 mL |
| Dried cranberries | 3/4 cup | 175 mL |
| Chopped pecans | 1/4 cup | 60 mL |

Preheat oven to 375°F (190°C). Cream butter and brown sugar in medium bowl. Add egg and vanilla. Beat until smooth.

Add next 5 ingredients. Beat on low until well combined.

Add cranberries and pecans. Stir. Drop, using 1 tbsp. (15 mL) for each, about 1 inch (2.5 cm) apart onto 2 greased cookie sheets. Flatten slightly with a fork. Bake on separate racks in oven for about 10 minutes, switching position of cookie sheets at halftime, until golden. Remove cookies from cookie sheets and place on wire racks to cool. Makes about 36 cookies.

*1 cookie: 76 Calories; 3.8 g Total Fat (1.1 g Mono, 0.3 g Poly, 1.8 g Sat); 12 mg Cholesterol; 9 g Carbohydrate; 1 g Fibre; 1 g Protein; 56 mg Sodium*

Pictured at left.

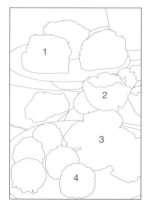

1. Pineapple Coconut Meringues, page 147
2. Strawberry Angel Cups, page 149
3. Oatmeal Cranberry Cookies, above
4. Date Crispies, page 146

Props courtesy of: Cherison Enterprises Inc.
Pier 1 Imports
Winners Stores

# Raspberry Parfait Fool

*Don't let the name fool you. With yogurt and non-fat pudding replacing the traditional whipped cream, this version of the classic English treat is a smart dessert choice!*

| | | |
|---|---|---|
| Box of instant non-fat vanilla pudding powder (4 serving size) | 1 | 1 |
| Milk | 1 cup | 250 mL |
| Vanilla yogurt | 1 cup | 250 mL |
| Lemon juice | 1 tbsp. | 15 mL |
| Grated lemon zest | 1 tsp. | 5 mL |
| Frozen (or fresh) whole raspberries | 1 1/2 cups | 375 mL |
| Flaked hazelnuts, toasted (see Tip, page 14) | 2 tbsp. | 30 mL |

Combine pudding powder and milk in medium bowl. Beat on low for about 2 minutes until smooth and thickened.

Add next 3 ingredients. Beat for 1 minute.

Fold in raspberries. Spoon into 4 serving dishes.

Sprinkle with hazelnuts. Serves 4.

*1 serving: 151 Calories; 4.0 g Total Fat (1.9 g Mono, 0.3 g Poly, 1.0 g Sat); 7 mg Cholesterol; 24 g Carbohydrate; 3 g Fibre; 6 g Protein; 366 mg Sodium*

# Date Crispies

*Another "I can't believe this is good for me" treat. Chewy and crispy, they're sure to satisfy all manner of cravings. Store them in the fridge—if they're still around after a few hours!*

| | | |
|---|---|---|
| Butter (or hard margarine) | 1 tbsp. | 15 mL |
| Chopped pitted dates | 1/2 cup | 125 mL |
| Granulated sugar | 1/4 cup | 60 mL |
| Large egg, fork-beaten | 1 | 1 |
| Crisp rice cereal | 1 1/2 cups | 375 mL |
| Salted, roasted sunflower seeds | 1/4 cup | 60 mL |

*(continued on next page)*

Melt butter in small saucepan on medium. Add next 3 ingredients. Cook for about 3 minutes, stirring constantly, until thickened. Remove from heat.

Add cereal and sunflower seeds. Stir. Let stand for about 10 minutes until cool enough to handle. Shape into 1 inch (2.5 cm) balls (see Note). Makes 18 crispies.

*1 crispy: 53 Calories; 1.8 g Total Fat (0.5 g Mono, 0.7 g Poly, 0.6 g Sat); 12 mg Cholesterol; 9 g Carbohydrate; 1 g Fibre; 1 g Protein; 53 mg Sodium*

Pictured on page 144.

**Note:** Coat hands lightly with cooking spray to prevent date mixture from sticking to them while forming into balls.

# Pineapple Coconut Meringues

*Tropical flavours abound! Sweet meringue with almonds and coconut tops a warm pineapple slice.*

| | | |
|---|---|---|
| Can of pineapple slices, drained | 14 oz. | 398 mL |
| Sliced natural almonds | 1/4 cup | 60 mL |
| Egg whites (large), room temperature | 2 | 2 |
| Vanilla extract | 1/2 tsp. | 2 mL |
| Granulated sugar | 2 tbsp. | 30 mL |
| Medium unsweetened coconut | 1/3 cup | 75 mL |
| Sliced natural almonds | 1/4 cup | 60 mL |
| Medium unsweetened coconut | 3 tbsp. | 50 mL |

Preheat oven to 400°F (205°C). Arrange 4 stacks of 2 pineapple slices in greased 9 inch (22 cm) pie plate. Sprinkle almonds over top. Set aside.

Beat egg whites in medium bowl until soft peaks form. Add vanilla. Add sugar 1 tbsp. (15 mL) at a time, beating constantly until stiff peaks form and sugar is dissolved.

Fold first amount of coconut and second amount of almonds into egg white mixture. Spoon onto pineapple.

Sprinkle with second amount of coconut. Bake in oven for about 10 minutes until meringue is golden. Serves 4.

*1 serving: 226 Calories; 12.2 g Total Fat (4.1 g Mono, 1.6 g Poly, 5.8 g Sat); 0 mg Cholesterol; 26 g Carbohydrate; 4 g Fibre; 5 g Protein; 32 mg Sodium*

Pictured on page 144.

# Chocolate Almond Puffs

*With just enough chocolate to make the worries of the day go away, these flourless puffs are crisp on the outside and soft on the inside.*

| | | |
|---|---|---|
| Ground almonds | 2 cups | 500 mL |
| Granulated sugar | 3/4 cup | 175 mL |
| Ground ginger | 1/4 tsp. | 1 mL |
| Salt | 1/8 tsp. | 0.5 mL |
| Egg whites (large), room temperature | 3 | 3 |
| Almond extract | 1/4 tsp. | 1 mL |
| Bittersweet chocolate baking squares (1 oz., 28 g, each), finely chopped | 4 | 4 |

Preheat oven to 350°F (175°C). Process first 4 ingredients in food processor (see Note) until well combined.

Add egg whites and extract. Process until mixture just starts to come together. Do not overmix. Transfer to medium bowl.

Add chocolate. Stir. Drop, using 1 tbsp. (15 mL) for each, about 1 inch (2.5 cm) apart onto 2 parchment paper-lined cookie sheets. Bake on separate racks in oven for about 12 minutes, switching position of cookie sheets at halftime, until tops puff up and bottoms are golden. Let stand on cookie sheets for about 5 minutes. Remove puffs and place on wire racks to cool. Makes about 30 puffs.

*1 puff: 75 Calories; 4.8 g Total Fat (2.0 g Mono, 0.8 g Poly, 1.1 g Sat); 0 mg Cholesterol; 8 g Carbohydrate; 1 g Fibre; 2 g Protein; 13 mg Sodium*

**Note:** If you don't have a food processor, an electric mixer can be used instead.

*fyi* Egg whites are high in protein, and contain none of the cholesterol found in egg yolks. Try using egg whites instead of whole eggs in baking, or in omelettes and other egg dishes. But if cholesterol is not a going concern for you, don't throw out your yolks just yet—although they do contain cholesterol, they also have many beneficial nutrients as well.

# Strawberry Angel Cups

*Individual pieces of heaven. The toasted cups put a unique spin on classic strawberry shortcake. For those who love the taste of orange liqueur, add just a little bit more!*

| | | |
|---|---|---|
| Slices of angel food cake, about 1/2 inch (12 mm) thick | 12 | 12 |
| Finely chopped fresh strawberries | 1 cup | 250 mL |
| Icing (confectioner's) sugar | 2 tbsp. | 30 mL |
| Orange liqueur | 1 tbsp. | 15 mL |
| Frozen light whipped topping, thawed | 3/4 cup | 175 mL |

Preheat oven to 350°F (175°C). Press cake slices into bottom and sides of 12 greased muffin cups. Bake on bottom rack in oven for about 15 minutes until bottoms are golden. Remove to wire rack to cool. Cups become crisp as they cool.

Combine next 3 ingredients in small bowl. Stir.

Spoon whipped topping into cups. Spoon strawberry mixture over topping. Makes 12 angel cups.

*1 angel cup: 99 Calories; 0.8 g Total Fat (trace Mono, 0.1 g Poly, 0.5 g Sat); 0 mg Cholesterol; 21 g Carbohydrate; 1 g Fibre; 2 g Protein; 213 mg Sodium*

Pictured on page 144.

 When choosing strawberries, indulge your urge to select only the reddest and most juicy-looking specimens—these brilliant berries don't continue to ripen after they're picked.

# Measurement Tables

Throughout this book measurements are given in Conventional and Metric measure. To compensate for differences between the two measurements due to rounding, a full metric measure is not always used. The cup used is the standard 8 fluid ounce. Temperature is given in degrees Fahrenheit and Celsius. Baking pan measurements are in inches and centimetres as well as quarts and litres. An exact metric conversion is given below as well as the working equivalent (Metric Standard Measure).

## Spoons

| Conventional Measure | Metric Exact Conversion Millilitre (mL) | Metric Standard Measure Millilitre (mL) |
|---|---|---|
| 1/8 teaspoon (tsp.) | 0.6 mL | 0.5 mL |
| 1/4 teaspoon (tsp.) | 1.2 mL | 1 mL |
| 1/2 teaspoon (tsp.) | 2.4 mL | 2 mL |
| 1 teaspoon (tsp.) | 4.7 mL | 5 mL |
| 2 teaspoons (tsp.) | 9.4 mL | 10 mL |
| 1 tablespoon (tbsp.) | 14.2 mL | 15 mL |

## Cups

| Conventional Measure | Metric Exact Conversion Millilitre (mL) | Metric Standard Measure Millilitre (mL) |
|---|---|---|
| 1/4 cup (4 tbsp.) | 56.8 mL | 60 mL |
| 1/3 cup (5 1/3 tbsp.) | 75.6 mL | 75 mL |
| 1/2 cup (8 tbsp.) | 113.7 mL | 125 mL |
| 2/3 cup (10 2/3 tbsp.) | 151.2 mL | 150 mL |
| 3/4 cup (12 tbsp.) | 170.5 mL | 175 mL |
| 1 cup (16 tbsp.) | 227.3 mL | 250 mL |
| 4 1/2 cups | 1022.9 mL | 1000 mL (1 L) |

## Dry Measurements

| Conventional Measure Ounces (oz.) | Metric Exact Conversion Grams (g) | Metric Standard Measure Grams (g) |
|---|---|---|
| 1 oz. | 28.3 g | 28 g |
| 2 oz. | 56.7 g | 57 g |
| 3 oz. | 85.0 g | 85 g |
| 4 oz. | 113.4 g | 125 g |
| 5 oz. | 141.7 g | 140 g |
| 6 oz. | 170.1 g | 170 g |
| 7 oz. | 198.4 g | 200 g |
| 8 oz. | 226.8 g | 250 g |
| 16 oz. | 453.6 g | 500 g |
| 32 oz. | 907.2 g | 1000 g (1 kg) |

## Oven Temperatures

| Fahrenheit (°F) | Celsius (°C) |
|---|---|
| 175° | 80° |
| 200° | 95° |
| 225° | 110° |
| 250° | 120° |
| 275° | 140° |
| 300° | 150° |
| 325° | 160° |
| 350° | 175° |
| 375° | 190° |
| 400° | 205° |
| 425° | 220° |
| 450° | 230° |
| 475° | 240° |
| 500° | 260° |

## Pans

| Conventional Inches | Metric Centimetres |
|---|---|
| 8x8 inch | 20x20 cm |
| 9x9 inch | 22x22 cm |
| 9x13 inch | 22x33 cm |
| 10x15 inch | 25x38 cm |
| 11x17 inch | 28x43 cm |
| 8x2 inch round | 20x5 cm |
| 9x2 inch round | 22x5 cm |
| 10x4 1/2 inch tube | 25x11 cm |
| 8x4x3 inch loaf | 20x10x7.5 cm |
| 9x5x3 inch loaf | 22x12.5x7.5 cm |

## Casseroles

| CANADA & BRITAIN | | UNITED STATES | |
|---|---|---|---|
| Standard Size Casserole | Exact Metric Measure | Standard Size Casserole | Exact Metric Measure |
| 1 qt. (5 cups) | 1.13 L | 1 qt. (4 cups) | 900 mL |
| 1 1/2 qts. (7 1/2 cups) | 1.69 L | 1 1/2 qts. (6 cups) | 1.35 L |
| 2 qts. (10 cups) | 2.25 L | 2 qts. (8 cups) | 1.8 L |
| 2 1/2 qts. (12 1/2 cups) | 2.81 L | 2 1/2 qts. (10 cups) | 2.25 L |
| 3 qts. (15 cups) | 3.38 L | 3 qts. (12 cups) | 2.7 L |
| 4 qts. (20 cups) | 4.5 L | 4 qts. (16 cups) | 3.6 L |
| 5 qts. (25 cups) | 5.63 L | 5 qts. (20 cups) | 4.5 L |

# Recipe Index

**152**

**154**

# S

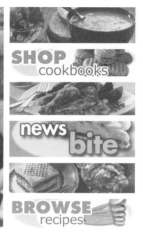

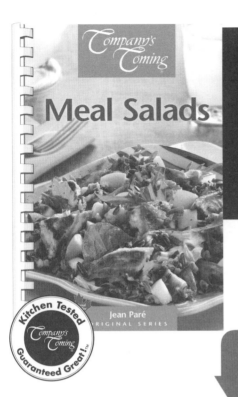

*Meal Salads* combines the crispness of fresh produce with the heartiness of grains, pastas, meats and cheeses, and get the best of both worlds—versatile dishes that are simple, fresh, tasty and filling.

# ⌠Try it

a sample recipe from *Meal Salads*

## Russian Wild Rice Salad

*Meal Salads*, Page 97

| | | |
|---|---|---|
| Water | 1 1/2 cups | 375 mL |
| Salt | 1/8 tsp. | 0.5 mL |
| Wild rice | 1/2 cup | 125 mL |
| Sour cream | 1/3 cup | 75 mL |
| Chopped fresh dill (or 3/4 tsp., 4 mL, dried) | 1 tbsp. | 15 mL |
| White wine vinegar | 1 tbsp. | 15 mL |
| Dry mustard | 1 tsp. | 5 mL |
| Coarsely ground pepper | 1/2 tsp. | 2 mL |
| Granulated sugar | 1/2 tsp. | 2 mL |
| Hot pepper sauce | 1/8 tsp. | 0.5 mL |
| Chopped fresh spinach leaves, lightly packed | 2 cups | 500 mL |
| Deli roast beef slices, cut into thin strips | 6 oz. | 170 g |
| Diced pickled beets | 2/3 cup | 150 mL |
| Diced English cucumber (with peel) | 1/2 cup | 125 mL |
| Finely diced pickled onions | 1 tbsp. | 15 mL |

Combine water and salt in small saucepan. Bring to a boil. Add rice. Stir. Reduce heat to medium-low.

Simmer, covered, for about 60 minutes, without stirring, until rice is tender. Drain any remaining liquid. Cool.

Whisk next 7 ingredients in large bowl.

Add remaining 5 ingredients and rice. Toss. Makes about 6 cups (1.5 L).

*1 cup (250 mL): 131 Calories; 3.5 g Total Fat (0.1 g Mono, 0.2 g Poly, 1.9 g Sat); 25 mg Cholesterol; 16 g Carbohydrate; 2 g Fibre; 9 g Protein; 286 mg Sodium*

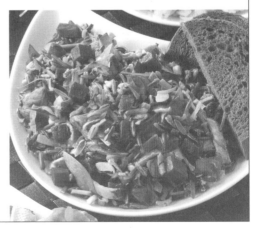

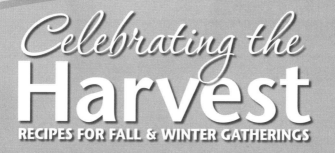

# Celebrating the
# Harvest
## RECIPES FOR FALL & WINTER GATHERINGS

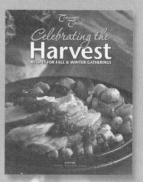

*Whether from the garden, farmers' market or supermarket, harvest ingredients display the bounty and beauty of nature. Entertain a crowd in style, or feed your family comfort food they'll not soon forget—with new delicious recipes that celebrate harvest ingredients. What a lovely way to get through the long fall and winter!*

SPECIAL OCCASION SERIES

# If you like what we've done with **cooking**, you'll **love** what we do with **crafts**!

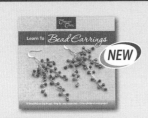 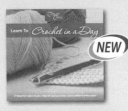 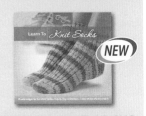

 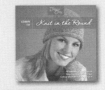 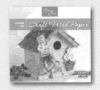 
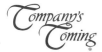